# Central Cholinergic
# Systems and Behaviour

# Central Cholinergic Systems and Behaviour

F. V. DeFEUDIS

Indiana University School of Medicine
Indianapolis, Indiana, U.S.A.

1974

## Academic Press

*London · New York · San Francisco*

ACADEMIC PRESS INC. (LONDON) LTD.
24/28 Oval Road, London NW1


*United States Edition published by*
ACADEMIC PRESS INC.
111 Fifth Avenue
New York, New York 10003

QP
921
P35
D43

Library of Congress Catalog Card Number: 74–5670
ISBN: 0–12–208750–Y

Text set in 11/12 pt. Monotype Baskerville, printed by letterpress,
and bound in Great Britain at The Pitman Press, Bath

# Foreword

More than three decades ago, Sir Henry Dale, in recognizing that acetyl-choline was acting as a chemical transmitter at certain peripheral synapses, pleaded that any suggestion of an analogous situation occurring at central synapses should not be made on a basis of suggestive analogy, but only in the light of direct and critically scrutinized evidence.

In the years that have passed since this advice was given we have made progress but it has been slow and hard won. We now have direct evidence that acetylcholine is a transmitter in the mammalian spinal cord and this evidence has withstood all scrutiny. Elsewhere in the central nervous system we have amassed a vast body of evidence to suggest that acetylcholine is likely to be an important transmitter at many sites but so far this evidence is incomplete and a definitive conclusion is not yet possible. Nevertheless, there is so much, and such a variety of indirect evidence pointing to acetylcholine as a transmitter in the brain that there is justification for considering what role this chemical is likely to play in central nervous function.

Dr. DeFeudis adopts a proper attitude in his consideration of the role of acetylcholine and has carefully pointed out the difficulties which still remain in interpretation and the many areas which are still open to controversy. He builds a persuasive case for cholinergic involvement in some of the more fundamental processes of central nervous functions and nicely presents and collates the available evidence so that the reader is smoothly guided through often conflicting evidence to a possible conclusion.

This book comes at an opportune time because so much data has recently accumulated on central cholinergic mechanisms but this has often been of an "isolated" nature with usually only hints of how it may fit into an overall cholinergic and non-cholinergic behavioural pattern. Dr. DeFeudis brings many of these experiments together and assesses them carefully in terms of overall central functional roles. Not everybody will agree with every conclusion that the author draws but the great wealth of data presented allows considered judgements to be made and an overall picture to emerge. It is encouraging that our knowledge of cholinergic systems has advanced to a stage where their implications and importance can be evaluated and it is a credit to the author that he has done this, but at the same time kept within the bounds of Dale's wise plea. Undoubtedly this work will stimulate further efforts to define and clarify the place of cholinergic systems in the brain.

*February 1974*                 J. F. MITCHELL, M.A., B.Sc., Ph.D., F.I.Biol.
                                Professor of Pharmacology
                                University of Bristol, England

# Preface

I am very grateful to the Academic Press (London) for giving me this opportunity to review studies about the possible involvement of central cholinergic systems in the regulation of animal behaviour. This review has served as a unique learning experience about an interesting subject. An attempt has been made to analyse and to integrate the significant data obtained by investigators who have employed a wide variety of scientific approaches. No effort has been made to balance the topics presented with regard to particular scientific disciplines, but rather, an emphasis has been placed on those approaches which have provided the best support for the development of certain concepts which seem necessary for making correlations between central cholinergic systems and behaviour. The various scientific approaches employed have been criticized in an effort to define some of the problems which should perhaps be attacked in future studies.

A principal point which has emerged from the analysis which is to be presented is that one can learn much about the central regulation of behaviour by studying the data that have been obtained from studies conducted on a proposed central neurotransmitter system. It is doubtful that different major conclusions regarding behaviour would have been achieved if studies about another proposed central transmitter system had been analysed.

Special thanks are due to Professor J. F. Mitchell both for helpful discussions about this work and for writing the Foreword, to Professor K. Krnjević for helpful discussions about this work and for providing facilities for photography and art work, and to Professor G. Pepeu, Professor J. W. Phillis and Professor J. C. Szerb for their criticism of an earlier draft of Chapter 6. My wife, Patricia, is also deserving of thanks for helpful discussions regarding psychological aspects of this work. I am also grateful to Mrs. Carol Lambert for assistance with the references, to Mr. N. Schestakowich and to members of the Medical Illustrations Department of Indiana University for assistance with the art work and photography, and to Mrs. Sandra Vasiliou for typing several drafts of the manuscript. The kind permission by other investigators and by publishers to reproduce the data which are presented in the tables and figures was also very much appreciated.

*February 1974*                                  F. V. DeFeudis, B.S., M.A., Ph.D.

# Contents

# Chapter 6

# Supporting Studies on the Central Release of Acetycholine

*for Patricia and Francis Roger*

# Chapter 1

# Introduction

Since a vast amount of information has now accumulated on cholinergic systems, it should not be surprising that a large body of evidence exists to support the association of central cholinergic mechanisms with behaviour. However, conclusive identification of cholinergic mechanisms responsible for specific behaviours has been difficult to achieve mainly because of the extensive anatomical and functional overlap of central pathways. Variations in experimental data caused by species differences, diurnal rhythms, housing conditions of experimental animals, maturation, and nutrition have also contributed to this problem. Also, many technological pitfalls have not yet been overcome. Nevertheless, many interesting studies have been conducted in this area, and some of the more pertinent ones will be reviewed herein. Good reviews of the early history of the biochemistry, physiology and pharmacology of the central cholinergic system have appeared (see e.g., Feldberg, 1945, 1950; Hebb and Krnjević, 1962; Quastel, 1962), and therefore early work will be presented here only when it is necessary for the development of a particular concept.

The striking symptoms displayed by human beings subjected to overdoses of cholinergic antagonists (e.g., atropine) or anticholinesterase agents (e.g. di-isopropyl-fluorophosphate; DFP) readily convince one that cholinergic systems are involved in a number of vital functions and in behaviour. However, it has not been established that these effects are "primary" in these cases, and hence these observations have not provided conclusive evidence for the existence of cholinergic regulation of behaviour. Administration of these agents to animals can cause convulsions and death, which adds further impetus to the notion that intact central cholinergic mechanisms are essential for an animal's normal function and behaviour. Furthermore, cholinergic agonists and antagonists, in smaller doses, affect both behavioural performance and EEG activity in man and other animals. Studies along these lines have led some investigators to suggest that the EEG can be "dissociated" from behaviour, though it seems more likely that EEG and behavioural

1

measurements have provided two separate methods for the analysis of brain function (see e.g. Wikler, 1952; Bradley and Elkes, 1957; Bradley and Nicholson, 1962).

In general, acetylcholine (ACh) and other cholinomimetic agents (e.g. carbachol) stimulate the cerebral cortex (and hippocampus) and cholinolytic agents (e.g. atropine) depress it, either by their direct actions on cortical neurones (Figs 1.1 and 1.2) or by their activation of

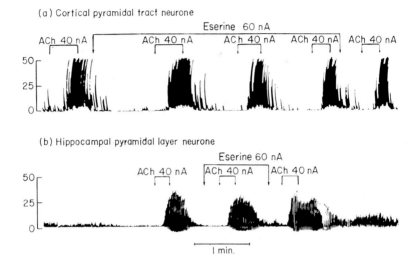

Fig. 1.1. Effects of iontophoretic applications of ACh and eserine on cortical and hippocampal neurones of an un-anaesthetized, "cerveau isolé" cat. Note the pronounced excitatory action of ACh which was slow in onset and of prolonged duration. Ordinates indicate firing frequency in counts/s; nA = *n*-Amps of iontophoretic current. Reproduced with permission from Salmoiraghi and Stefanis (1967).

diffuse pathways which project to, and innervate, these neurones. But, recently good evidence has been provided for an inhibitory action of ACh on a system of intra-cortical neurones (see e.g. Phillis and York, 1968) which had previously been described by histochemical methods (Krnjević and Silver, 1965; see Fig. 2.4). All studies of the effects of anti-cholinesterase (anti-ChE) agents on central neurones are at most only speculative since it is well known that these agents also inhibit cellular respiration and enzymes other than ChE (e.g. Brooks *et al.*, 1949; Michaelis *et al.*, 1949). Also, in some studies, such large doses of cholinomimetic or cholinolytic agents have been used that peripheral actions (e.g. cardiovascular reflexes) could have contributed appreciably to the effects which were monitored in the CNS.

In several reviews the possible functional roles of central cholinergic systems have been described in some detail using data obtained in histochemical, biochemical, pharmacological, and behavioural studies (see e.g. Feldberg, 1950, 1954; Holmstedt, 1959; Hebb and Krnjević, 1962; Carlton, 1963, 1969; DeRobertis, 1964; Eccles, 1964; Krnjević, 1965a,

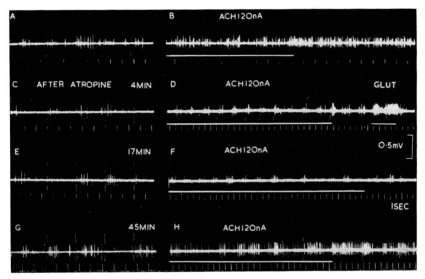

FIG. 1.2. Muscarinic character of a cerebral cortical neurone of cat's brain. Control record shows characteristic repetitive discharge after single shocks to ventroposterolateral thalamic nucleus (A) and excitatory effect of ACh applied for 38 s (B). Records *C* and *D* were taken 4 min. after the end of a 2 min. application of atropine (80 nA); ACh excitation was blocked, though L-glutamate had its usual excitatory effect. Full responses had not returned at 17 min. (*E,F*), even though ACh was applied for 54 seconds. Recovery occurred at about 45 min. after the end of the release of atropine, as shown by reappearance of ACh sensitivity and repetitive discharges (*G,H*). Horizontal lines below records indicate last part of ACh application. Reproduced with permission from Krnjević (1964).

1967, 1969; Whittaker, 1965; Votava, 1967; Karczmar, 1967; Koelle, 1969; Phillis, 1970; Hebb, 1970; Pradhan and Dutta, 1971; Deutsch, 1971). Although not any one of these approaches can, in itself, provide conclusive evidence for the existence of cholinergic pathways, some association between central cholinergic mechanisms and behaviour now seems likely. Several major functional roles for central cholinergic systems have emerged. For example, cholinergic elements appear to be involved in the function of non-specific, reticulo-cortical pathways which are responsible for cortical arousal, and hence for effective cortical function and behaviour (see Chapters 2, 5 and 6; Fig. 2.1). Other evidence has been provided for a link between central cholinergic and adrenergic systems in the mediation of behavioural arousal, and for the existence of an inhibitory cholinergic system in behavioural regulation (see e.g. Russell *et al.*, 1961; Carlton, 1963, 1969; Reeves, 1966; Russell, 1969; Fibiger *et al.*, 1970; Chapters 2, 5 and 6). Central cholinergic systems also seem to play a role in motor reflexes and postural mechanisms since the axons of cholinergic lower motoneurones innervate skeletal muscle and spinal Renshaw cells, and since cholinergic elements are associated with extrapyramidal, reticular, and cerebellar functions (see Chapter 3). Since direct injections of cholinergic agents into nuclei of the extrapyramidal system cause tremor, catalepsy and "circling" behaviours (e.g. Mennear, 1965; Connor *et al.*, 1966a; Baker *et al.*, 1967a; Costall *et al.*, 1972), and since anti-cholinergic agents have been useful in the treatment of Parkinsonism, it seems likely that behaviours regulated by extrapyramidal function are produced, at least in part, by cholinergic mechanisms (see Chapter 3). Cholinergic innervation of the cerebellum, though diffuse, has implicated this system in the central control of motor integration and coordination (see Chapter 3). The relationship between acetylcholine (ACh) and central autonomic mechanisms has stemmed from studies on: (1) the release of anti-diuretic hormone (Chang *et al.*, 1937, a, b, c; Huang, 1938; Pickford, 1939); (2) respiratory mechanisms (Dikshit, 1934a, b, c; Gesell *et al.*, 1943); and, (3) thermoregulation (Henderson and Wilson, 1936). Recently, many studies have been conducted on the possible roles of central cholinergic systems in relation to homeostatic functions and motivated behaviours (see Chapters 4 and 5).

Further studies have indicated that central cholinergic mechanisms may be involved in emotionality, learning and memory (see Chapter 5). In this regard, Feldberg and Sherwood (1954) showed that "catatonic-like" states could be produced in experimental animals by intra-ventricular injections of DFP, eserine, or large quantities of ACh, itself, and earlier Sherwood (1952) had interrupted catatonic stupor in some schizophrenic patients with intra-ventricular injections of a preparation of "true" ChE. These studies, along with others which showed that catatonic behaviours could be produced by electrical stimulation of the diencephalon (Hess, 1954), led to the suggestion that the behavioural functions of structures bordering the cerebral ventricles (e.g. hypothalamus, caudate nucleus) might be subserved by cholinergic mechanisms. Also, some anti-ChE agents have been shown to exert psychotomimetic effects in man (see e.g. DeBoor, 1956; Longo and Scotti de Carlos, 1968), which adds strength to the view that cholinergic mechanisms may be involved in mental functions. In this regard, it is noteworthy that lysergic acid diethylamide (LSD) treatment causes many "atropine-like" effects in man (e.g. hypertension, hyperthermia, mydriasis; see Pfeiffer, 1959), and that atropine and some of its derivatives can produce psychotomimetic effects in man (Forrer, 1951; Miller, 1956; Ostfeld *et al.*, 1959; Giarman and Pepeu, 1962; Abood and Biel, 1962; Ostfeld and Aruguete, 1962; White, 1966).

On the basis of the above-mentioned studies, and others to be discussed in this monograph, it seems reasonable to suspect that central cholinergic mechanisms may be involved in altered emotional and mental states of man. However, it cannot be over-emphasized that in many of the studies performed to date cholinomimetic or cholinolytic agents have been administered systemically, and that this has led to many problems in both interpreting and reproducing the observed behavioural effects. Although, in some cases, this problem has been overcome to some extent by using drug congeners which do not enter the brain, many of the data obtained on cholinergic mechanisms of behaviour will require future reinterpretation. Some of the difficulties encountered when using systemic injections are due to: (1) lack of, or slow entry of injected substances into the CNS due to "blood-brain barrier" mechanisms; (2) actions of the injected agents at peripheral sites which can modify cerebral activity by "secondary" or "reflex" actions; (3) metabolism, or inactivation (e.g. by "binding") of the agents administered; (4) dilution, by body fluids, of the agents administered; (5) local effects of the agents on vascular mechanisms which can lead to alterations in cellular metabolism (see e.g. Hebb and Krnjević, 1962). Due to these factors, experiments in which intra-carotid injections of ACh or cholinolytic agents (e.g. DFP) have been shown to affect excitability of the brain or to cause "discrete" behavioural patterns (e.g. Bremer, 1937; Essig *et al.*, 1950; Himwich *et al.*, 1950) have not provided strong evidence for the existence of central cholinergic mechanisms (see §3.5). Evidence obtained by using methods based on intra-cerebral injection, brain lesioning, ACh release, histochemistry and iontophoresis, though also subject to much criticism, seems to have provided more conclusive support for an association between central cholinergic mechanisms and behaviour. In any case, in order to gain insight into the complex mechanisms of behaviour it is necessary to derive "molar conceptions of neural action" (Hebb, 1949), and this can only be accomplished by integrating data obtained with a wide variety of scientific approaches. Therefore, an effort will be made to integrate data obtained from various disciplines in order to define further the roles which central cholinergic systems may play in the regulation of behaviour.

*Chapter 2*

# Cholinergic Roles in Consciousness

## 2.1 Arousal: Reticular-Activating System

"Arousal" may be divided operationally into two categories for purposes of discussion: (1) "cortical arousal" or "EEG activation" (desynchronization) which characterizes the "waking state" and the state of "paradoxical" (r.e.m.) sleep of the animal; (2) "behavioural arousal" or increased sense of awareness of the animal, i.e. increased sensitivity to incoming stimuli, which seems to be the functional substrate for emotional and motivational phenomena. More generally, arousal may be thought of as a system of interrelated phenomena which is involved in maintaining the conscious state of an organism—a system as essential to life as "sleep" and "wakefulness", which may indeed be its component parts. Many cerebrospinal structures are associated with the arousal mechanism (see Figs 2.1, 2.2, and 2.3). This is a "diffuse" system with many peripheral inputs, including those from ascending spinal tracts, from the brain stem, itself, and from specific sensory pathways (i.e. via the spinal and cranial nerves). All of this information is channelled ultimately into a final common pathway which emanates from the brain stem reticular formation ("reticular-activating system") and projects, via the non-specific thalamic nuclei and hypothalamus, to the cerebral cortex, hippocampus, and other structures to produce neocortical and limbic activation (see e.g. Moruzzi and Magoun, 1949; Fig. 2.1). Descending reticular systems also play roles in the arousal mechanism (Figs 2.2 and 2.3). Limbic activation (e.g. activation of the hippocampus) seems to occur predominantly by pathways emanating from hypothalamic structures since the hippocampal EEG can be activated in cats which have been transected at levels rostral to the midbrain, while neocortical activation seems to occur by pathways which traverse the mesencephalic reticular formation (e.g. Kawamura *et al.*, 1961; Kawamura and Domino, 1968; see below). Although consciousness may be governed by the whole brain, the reticular formation and the

7

non-specific thalamocortical system are perhaps its main anatomical components (e.g. Jasper, 1958). It should be noted that although central cholinergic systems appear to be involved in arousal, other possible transmitter systems (e.g. those which may utilize noradrenaline, dopamine or glutamate) may also play important roles (see below, and Chapter 6). It seems possible now to make an attempt to correlate

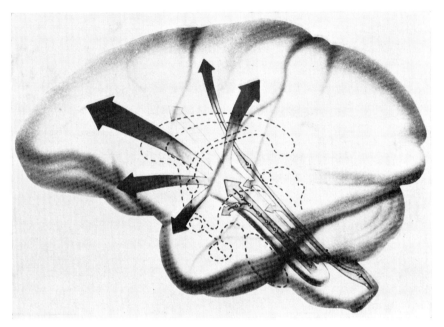

Fig. 2.1. Phantom drawing of human brain depicting the reticular-activating system. Lemniscal (classical) sensory pathways are shown ascending from spinal and brain stem levels to the somesthetic receiving area of the cortex and giving off collaterals into the brain stem reticular formation. The reticular formation is shown containing extra-lemniscal ascending projections which influence the hypothalamus and which diverge at the level of the thalamus to distribute impulses diffusely throughout all areas of the cortex. Stimulation of the reticular-activating system initiates and sustains generalized electrical and behavioural activation of the nervous system. Reproduced with permission from Magoun (1954).

studies performed on cholinergic mechanisms with regard to: (1) gross and microscopic structures of the brain; (2) brain-lesioned animals; (3) specific sensory systems; (4) iontophoretic effects; (5) neocortical and limbic EEG activation; (6) behavioural changes produced by various pharmacological agents; and (7) release of ACh from brain regions.

Bradley and Elkes (1953) first showed that systemic injections of di-isopropyl-fluorophosphate (DFP) or eserine into sleeping or resting animals caused EEG activation and behavioural arousal (see also Bradley *et al.*, 1953). However, since EEG activation also occurs during paradoxical sleep, behavioural arousal does not always follow EEG arousal. Using intra-carotid injections of ACh, Rinaldi and Himwich (1955a, b) provided evidence that cholinergic mechanisms of the

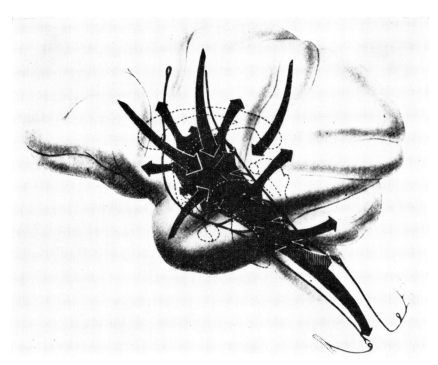

Fig. 2.2. Schematic representation of the relations of the reticular core of the brain stem (*black*) with other systems of the brain. Collaterals are shown entering the reticular core from long sensory and motor tracts (*thin lines*) and from cerebral hemispheres. The core acts in turn on cerebral and cerebellar cortices (*upward-directed arrows*) and associated structures, on spinal cord (*long, downward-directed arrow*), and on central sensory relays (*striped arrows*). Reproduced with permission from Worden and Livingston (1961).

mesencephalic reticular formation (MRF) might be involved in cortical arousal, since the effects of the injected ACh were not altered in "cerveau isolé" preparations (see also Bovet and Longo, 1956). Although it has been known for a long time that electrical stimulation of a variety of peripheral afferent systems, or of the brain stem reticular formation, can cause a generalized arousal response (e.g. Rheinberger and Jasper, 1937; Moruzzi and Magoun, 1949), good evidence for a direct action of

ACh on this system is lacking. In the above studies of Rinaldi and Himwich, visual and olfactory pathways which remain functional in "cerveau isolé" preparations could have been activated by the injected ACh and this could have led to cortical arousal. The effects on these cells of intra-carotid administration of ACh could also have been related to

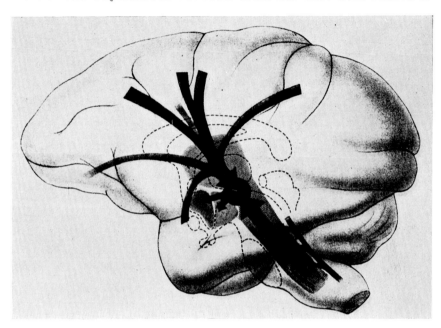

Fig. 2.3. Phantom drawing of human brain depicting ascending sensory, descending corticofugal and hypothalamic outflow. Classical (lemniscal) sensory pathways (*interrupted*) can be seen passing collateral projections into the brain stem reticular formation. Descending corticofugal projections arise from frontal eye fields, somatosensory cortex, paraoccipital region, superior gyrus of the temporal lobe and from more medial regions of the orbital surface and cingulate gyrus. Corticofugal projections converge in the same general regions of the brain stem which are occupied by extra-lemniscal ascending projections. Convergences of sensory, motor and visceral projections relate intimately to subthalamic and hypothalamic regions which appear to play a key role in the regulation of goal-directed behaviours. Reproduced with permission from Livingston (1955).

vasomotor changes (see e.g. Bovet and Longo, 1956). However, in this connection, more recent studies have indicated that some brainstem reticular cells appear to be cholinoceptive (Bradley and Wolstencroft, 1962, 1965; Salmoiraghi and Steiner, 1963; Bradley *et al.*, 1966; Yamamoto, 1967; see Phillis, 1970).

Histochemical findings, based on AChE staining, have supported the concept of a cholinergically-mediated arousal system. A continuous system of cholinergic fibres appears to project to the hypothalamus, basal ganglia and cerebral cortex from the brainstem (Shute and Lewis, 1963; 1967; Krnjević and Silver, 1965). It has also been shown that AChE staining is confined mainly to deeper neocortical cells (Krnjević and

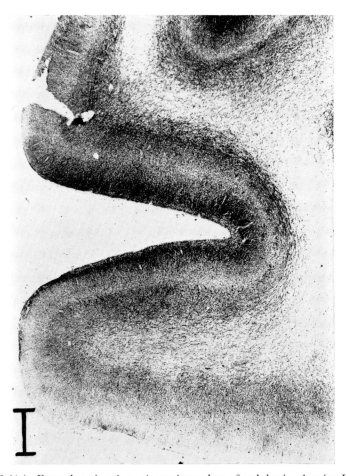

FIG. 2.4(a). Frontal section through cruciate sulcus of cat's brain, showing U-fibres and the deep and superficial zones of staining; the latter is particularly well developed in the walls of the sulcus. Black dots at the outer margin of the deep zone are stained pyramidal cells. Thiocholine method. Scale: 1·0 mm. Reproduced with permission from Krnjević and Silver (1965).

Silver, 1965; see Fig. 2.4) which are primarily excited by iontophoreti-cally-administered ACh (Krnjević and Phillis, 1963a, b, c; Krnjević, 1965a, b). In their study of the effects of cortical undercutting in the cat, Hebb *et al.* (1963) concluded, from data on AChE and choline acetylase

(ChAc) activities, that cholinergic fibres innervating cortical cells may project from distant cortical regions or from deeper nuclei. The AChE content of pyramidal cells in layer V of the cortex was high, which supported the findings obtained in iontophoretic studies (see above); AChE staining indicated also that subcortical cells of the corpus striatum and precommissural septum, as well as fibres from adjacent gyri, project to the cerebral cortex (see also Krnjević and Silver, 1965; Figs 2.4 and 2.5).

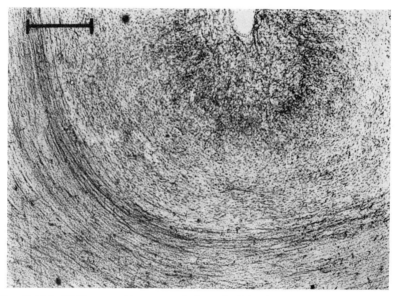

Fɪɢ. 2.4(b). U-fibres curving around the splenial sulcus in a cat's brain. Thio-choline method. Scale: 0·5 mm. Reproduced with permission from Krnjević and Silver (1965).

The above evidence, along with that provided by studies in which it was shown that cortical ACh release was increased during neocortical activation (e.g. Mitchell, 1963, 1966; Kanai and Szerb, 1965; Celesia and Jasper, 1966; Szerb, 1967; see Chapter 6), supported further the idea that arousal is mediated, at least in part, by cholinergic mechanisms. It has also been reported that cortical ACh release is reduced in chloralose-anaesthetized animals and that it can be reduced further by increasing the depth of anaesthesia (MacIntosh and Oborin, 1953; Mitchell, 1963). This reduction, by chloralose, of spontaneously-released ACh may be related to its depressant effect on the reticular formation which would decrease the level of cortical arousal (Moruzzi and Magoun, 1949; Bremer and Stoupel, 1959). Chloralose prevents both behavioural and EEG arousal while atropine (*d,l*-hyoscyamine) prevents only the latter, a difference which might be explained by considering the direct action of chloralose on brain stem mechanisms.

Recent evidence has indicated that stimulation of specific sensory pathways (e.g. visual and auditory), like stimulation of peripheral

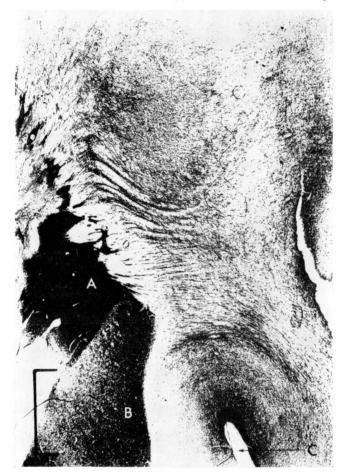

FIG. 2.5. Frontal section of cat's brain showing stained fibres from the putamen radiating towards the lateral cortex. Note that the lateral amygdaloid nucleus shows some activity and that U-fibres around the rhinal fissure link neocortex and paleo-cortex. (A) Putamen; (B) lateral amygdaloid nucleus; (C), rinal fissure. Thiocholine method. Scale 0·5 mm. Reproduced with permission from Krnjević and Silver (1965).

nerves and the reticular formation, causes mainly a widespread release of ACh from many areas of the cortex (Phillis, 1968a; Bartolini *et al.*, 1972), while in other experiments (Collier and Mitchell, 1966, 1967; Hemsworth and Mitchell, 1969) increases in ACh release were found to be greatest from cortical receiving areas associated with the stimulated pathway (see Chapter 6). Perhaps an attempt should be made to correlate these conflicting sets of data in order to provide a general hypothesis concerning cortical ACh release. It is suggested that increases in the release of ACh may be caused by any type of stimulation which

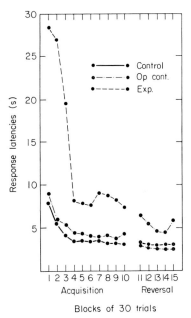

Blocks of 30 trials

FIG. 2.6. Effects of crystalline implants of carbachol (0·5–1·0 $\mu$g) into the MRF on acquisition and performance of escape (shuttle-box) responses in the rat. Cholinergic stimulation and test trials were given at 72-h intervals; 8 rats received bilateral cholinergic stimulation of the MRF 5 min. before each 15-trial test; 8 rats served as unoperated controls and 8 more as operated controls. Note that latencies were increased by carbachol during both acquisition and at asymptote and that implant-produced lesions did not affect these escape responses. Reproduced with permission from Grossman (1966b).

alters an organism's sense of awareness to incoming stimuli and that these may be mediated, at least in part, by the non-specific, reticulo-cortical system. Specific sensory relay nuclei of the thalamus (e.g. those of visual and auditory systems), as well as other thalamic nuclei, are likely to have projections to the reticulo-cortical system, perhaps via the intralaminar and midline nuclei (Nauta and Whitlock, 1954), and hence could be components of the arousal system (see Figs 2.1, 2.2 and 2.3). This seems possible even though extra-thalamic pathways from midbrain to cortex are known to exist (e.g. Starzl *et al.*, 1951). One could also argue that increases in specific sensory input causes an altered state of consciousness (awareness) in the animal and therefore should increase the diffuse release of ACh. This may indeed be a major function of the arousal system, as defined. This hypothesis receives some support from the studies of Phillis *et al.* (1968) in which it was shown that the release of ACh from some thalamic areas was increased by stimulation of peripheral nerves (see Chapter 6). Also relevant to this hypothesis is the finding of Jasper and Koyama (1969) that low-frequency electrical stimulation of the mesial thalamic nuclei (thalamic recruiting system) evoked a release of ACh from the cortex (see Chapter 6). It is well known

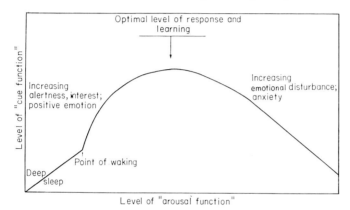

Fig. 2.7. Graph demonstrating the relationship in an animal between the effectiveness of "cue function" (which guides behaviour) and the level of "arousal function" (a measure of non-specific cortical bombardment). Note that without a foundation of arousal, the cue function cannot exist. Reproduced with permission from Hebb (1955).

from early work that stimulation of the mesial thalamic nuclei can affect EEG arousal elicited by ascending reticular volleys, and that reticular impulses which produce EEG and behavioural arousal may be mediated by a diffuse thalamic projection to the cortex (Dempsey and Morrison, 1942, 1943; Moruzzi and Magoun, 1949; Jasper, 1949; Starzl and Magoun, 1951; Jasper *et al.*, 1952).

Another line of evidence which supports the hypothesis that cholinergic mechanisms might be involved in arousal stems from behavioural experiments performed with intra-cerebral injection techniques. Injections of ACh or other cholinergic agents (e.g. carbachol) directly into the mesencephalic or thalamic reticular formation of the rat produced reversible behavioural changes in both appetitive and aversive test situations (e.g. Grossman, 1966b; Grossman and Grossman, 1966; Grossman and Peters, 1966; Grossman, 1968; see Fig. 2.6 and Chapter 5). These workers concluded that cholinergic stimulation increased markedly the animal's responsiveness to sensory stimulation; effects obtained with adrenergic agents were of opposite trend. These results indicated that cholinergic reticular mechanisms might be involved in behavioural arousal which is necessary for learning processes. However, marked species differences do seem to exist. For example, in cats, cholinergic stimulation of similar brain structures induced sleep, while

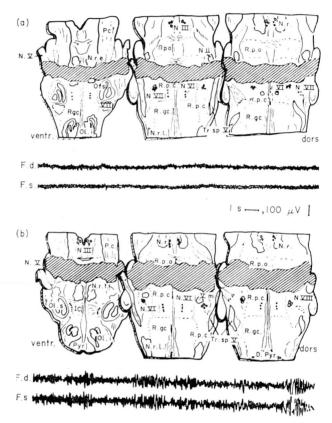

FIG. 2.8. (a). Mid-pontine, pre-trigeminal section of the brain stem. Desynchronized cortical EEG activity (arousal) was obtained by separation of the caudal synchronizing structures from the arousal system which is located just rostral to the transection. (b) Rostro-pontine transection of the brain stem. The EEG was synchronized since the caudal part of the arousal system was destroyed by the lesion. Reproduced with permission from Batini *et al.*, (1958).

adrenergic stimulation caused increases in arousal and alertness (Hernández Peón *et al.*, 1963a, b; 1965).

## 2.2 Sleep-Wakefulness: Neocortical and Limbic Activation

The principal manifestations of the arousal mechanism may be considered to be: (1) slow-wave sleep (characterized by EEG synchroniza-

tion); (2) fast-wave (r.e.m.) sleep (characterized by EEG desynchronization); and (3) wakefulness (characterized by EEG desynchronization).
The various phases of sleep and wakefulness should be considered as
parts of a continuum, rather than as isolated states. The level of arousal
of an animal is decreased markedly during slow-wave and fast-wave
sleep, and is increased during wakefulness (see Fig. 2.7). It should be
noted, when studying the literature on sleep and wakefulness, that
many of the earlier studies (e.g. those of Bradley and Elkes, 1953) were

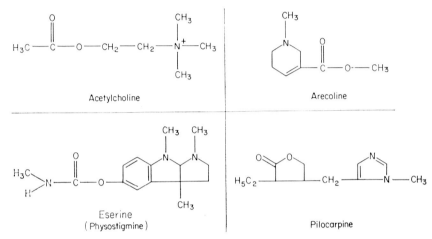

FIG. 2.9. Chemical structures of some predominantly muscarinic cholinergic
agonists. Reproduced with permission from Domino *et al.*, (1968).

interpreted without a knowledge of the existence of fast-wave (paradoxical) sleep. This type of sleep was described later (Dement, 1958;
Jouvet, 1961, 1965). Behavioural changes associated with "initial"
EEG activation seem to be clearly related to arousal while some sleep
states perhaps involve the "hypnogenic circuit" postulated by Hernández-Peón and colleagues (1963a, b; 1965).

In early studies, Dikshit (1934c, 1935) showed that intra-hypothalamic or intra-ventricular injections of ACh (1–5 $\mu$g) produced "sleeplike" states in cats in 10–30 minutes which lasted for a few hours. ACh
administration can also produce drowsy states in humans (Hoffer, 1954).
Considerable pharmacological evidence exists to support the central
cholinergic mediation of neocortical and limbic EEG activation,
behavioural arousal and sleep (see e.g. reviews by Killam, 1962;
Stümpf, 1965; Longo, 1966). Much of this evidence has been obtained
using drugs which potentiate, mimic, or inhibit the actions of ACh (e.g.
Knapp and Domino, 1962; Villarreal and Domino, 1964; Domino *et*

*al.*, 1965, 1967, 1968; Yamamoto and Domino, 1965, 1967; see Figs 2.9, 2.10, 2.12, 2.13). Studies on the central release of ACh conducted in relation to levels of cortical arousal, have also contributed considerably to our knowledge of mechanisms of sleep and wakefulness (see Chapter 6). The diffuse cortical release of ACh caused by reticular activation appears to be associated with mechanisms of sleep and wakefulness. Theoretically, as suggested by Krnjević (1965b), the level of cortical arousal may be related to the amount of ACh released from cholinergic fibres which ascend from subcortical structures to innervate deep pyramidal cells of the cerebral cortex. However, a shortcoming exists in relating data obtained in many release studies to "normal" mechanisms of sleep and wakefulness since these have been carried out with

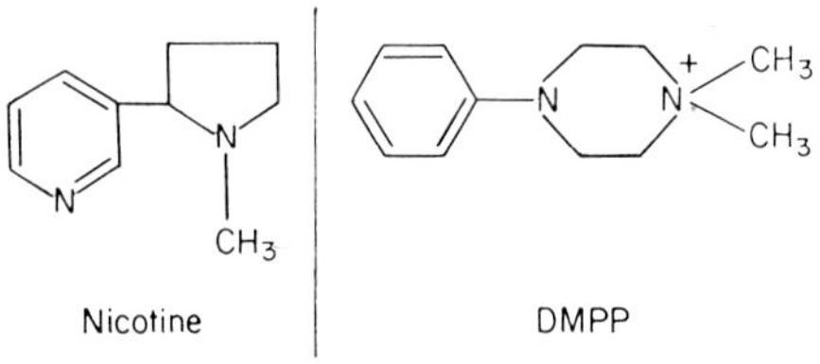

Nicotine            DMPP

FIG. 2.10. Chemical structures of two predominantly nicotinic (ganglionic) cholinergic agonists; *DMPP* = 1,1-dimethyl-4-phenylpiperidinium. Reproduced with permission from Domino *et al.*, (1968).

anaesthetized animals (but see Collier and Mitchell, 1967; Beani *et al.*, 1968; Jasper and Tessier, 1971; and Chapter 6). Evidence has indicated that impulses in ascending specific sensory pathways (lemniscal system) persist while those in the reticular system tend to be blocked during anaesthesia (e.g. French *et al.*, 1953; Arduini and Arduini, 1954; Killam and Killam, 1958).

Studies conducted by Pepeu and Mantegazzini (1964) have provided good evidence that the ACh content of the cerebral cortex is associated with sleep and wakefulness. Midbrain hemisections of cats produced EEG synchronization ("sleeping cortex") which was correlated with increases in cortical ACh content, while mid-pontine, pre-trigeminal lesions caused EEG desynchronization ("awake cortex") which was correlated with decreases in ACh content. By making both lesions in the same cat it was shown that the ACh content was always greater in the "sleeping" than in the "awake" cortex (see Table 1). These workers suggested that the increases in cortical ACh which occurred during EEG synchronization may have been due to ACh accumulation in the terminals of cortical afferent fibres and/or to its increase in some cortical neurones. These findings were supported by further studies which revealed that ACh was released to a greater extent from "awake" than from "sleeping" cortex (Bartolini and Pepeu, 1967; see Chapter 6; Fig. 6.3). It may be concluded from these studies that ACh content and release in the cortex are inversely related and that both are altered by changes in the level of cortical activity. With regard to the underlying physiological mechanism, it is known that midbrain hemi-section causes sleep ipsilateral to the lesion by decreasing subcortical afferent

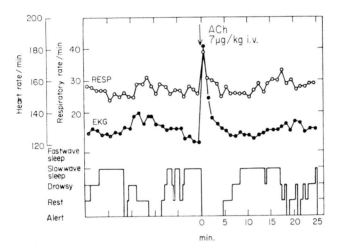

Fig. 2.11. Effects of an intravenous injection of a large dose of ACh to a sleeping cat bearing chronic indwelling brain electrodes in the amygdalae and hippocampi and bipolar ball electrodes on the posterior sigmoid gyrus. Note that ACh caused marked increases in respiration and heart rate and a transient period of EEG activation and behavioural arousal which lasted for about 4 minutes. Reproduced with permission from Yamamoto and Domino (1967).

input to the cortex (Cordeau and Mancia, 1958), and that mid-pontine, pre-trigeminal lesions cause EEG desynchronization to be maintained due to "tonic" afferent impulses from the rostral pons (Batini *et al.*, 1958, 1959a, b; see Fig. 2.8). Although the relationship between ACh content and release, on the one hand, and state of activation of the cortex, on the other, may seem simple, the use of pharmacological agents (e.g. atropine, neostigmine) during release studies has revealed that it is quite complex (e.g. Celesia and Jasper, 1966) and has led to several interesting concepts about the "dissociation" of the EEG from ACh release, and from behaviour (see § 2.3, Chapter 6; Figs 6.1 and 6.2).

Further studies on the possible cholinergic mechanisms underlying sleep and wakefulness have been focused on elucidating the nature of the

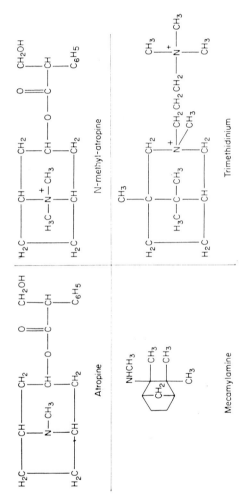

Fig. 2.12. Chemical structures of two muscarinic cholinergic antagonists (atropine and N-methylatropine) and two nicotinic (ganglionic) cholinergic antagonists (mecamylamine and trimethidinium). Reproduced with permission from Domino *et al.*, (1968).

TABLE 1. Acetylcholine content (nanograms of the chloride per 100 mg fresh tissue) of the cerebral cortex and caudate nucleus in mid-pontine pre-trigeminal preparations from cats with midbrain hemisections. Reproduced with permission from Pepeu and Mantegazzini (1964).

| Cat. No. | Frontal area | | Parietal area | | Occipital area | | Caudate nucleus | |
|---|---|---|---|---|---|---|---|---|
| | Control | Hemi-sected | Control | Hemi-sected | Control | Hemi-sected | Control | Hemi-sected |
| 1 | 109·2 | 160·1 | 87·2 | 207·6 | 72·0 | 189·0 | 510·2 | 546·2 |
| 2 | 71·6 | 194·9 | 96·8 | 187·2 | 65·8 | 231·8 | 363·6 | 413·1 |
| 3 | 50·6 | 174·4 | 103·8 | 147·6 | 57·2 | 121·2 | 290·1 | 381·7 |
| 4 | 165·9 | 188·8 | 91·5 | 195·3 | 103·2 | 230·7 | 328·1 | 372·6 |
| 5 | 89·6 | 141·8 | 77·9 | 167·0 | 73·5 | 115·0 | 520·0 | 560·0 |
| Mean ± S.E. | 93·3 ± 20·0 | 172·0 ± 9·8 | 91·4 ± 3·7 | 180·9 ± 10·6 | 74·3 ± 7·7 | 177·5 ± 25·5 | 402·4 ± 47·0 | 454·7 ± 40·3 |
| | $p < ·01$ | | $p < ·001$ | | $p < ·01$ | | Nonsignificant | |
| Average increase | 73·9% | | 98·3% | | 138·9% | | 13·0% | |
| After injection of DL-DOPA | | | | | | | | |
| 6 | 104·0 | 75·4 | 75·6 | 119·3 | 75·0 | 93·9 | 367·7 | 390·2 |
| 7 | 89·9 | 92·4 | 75·0 | 88·6 | 81·8 | 70·1 | 353·3 | 375·0 |

receptor(s) involved. Considerable evidence exists to su
both muscarinic and nicotinic receptors in neocortical a
Mikhelson, 1961; Valdman, 1961, 1963; Denisenko, 1
enok, 1962; Knapp and Domino, 1962; Yamamoto and I
For example, it is well known that large systemic doses of
neocortical activation elicited by several different stimu
(e.g. see Domino and Hudson, 1958; White and Boyaj\
and Daigneault, 1959). Pre-treatment of cats with atro
EEG activation produced by muscarinic agonists (e.g. A
eserine (physostigmine), pilocarpine; Fig. 2.9), but onl
caused by nicotinic agonists (e.g. DMPP, nicotine, s
nicotine-induced hippocampal theta-wave activity wa

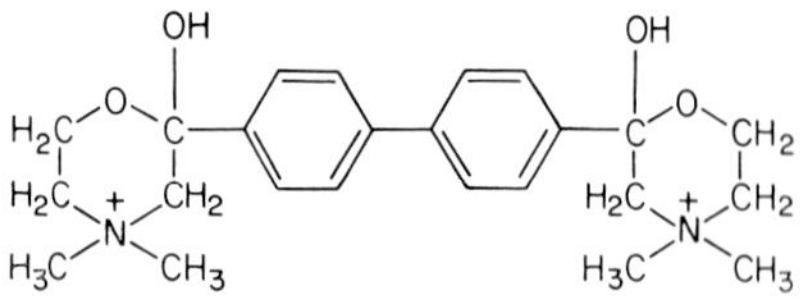

Fig. 2.13. Chemical structure of hemicholinium-3 (HC-3), an ag
ACh synthesis. Reproduced with permission from Domino *et al.* (19

atropine (Domino, 1966, 1968; Domino *et al.*, 1968).
bearing chronically-implanted electrodes, Yamamoto
(1967) showed that intravenous injections of ACh (7
neocortical and limbic EEG activation and behaviour.
that these actions were prevented by pretreatment of th
muscarinic antagonists (e.g. atropine and N-methylatr
0·3 mg/kg, i.v.; see Figs 2.11 and 2.12), but not by nico
antagonists (Fig. 2.12). It was suggested that the terr
responsible for neocortical activation might involve musc
a view which is consistent with other data obtained wit
and release methods (see e.g. Krnjević, 1964, 1965a, b; D
1969; Chapter 6; Fig. 1.2), and that muscarinic, and to
nicotinic, receptors might be involved in neocortical a
activation. According to Domino *et al.*, (1968), injection
or eserine awaken cats from sleep, but after a short time
by drowsiness and then fast-wave sleep. These pha
evoked arousal responses were blocked by anti-muscarin
N-methyl-atropine (which exerts mainly peripheral
effects) antagonized EEG activation caused by ACh, but
by other muscarinic or nicotinic agonists (Domino *et a*
these studies, it was concluded that the gross behaviour o

EEG changes in the neocortex which were produced by low doses of these agents.

Hemicholinium-3 (HC-3; Fig. 2.13) has been used to study the cholinergic nature of mechanisms of EEG activation since this agent is known to inhibit ACh synthesis (and hence, to reduce tissue ACh content) both *in vivo* and *in vitro*, perhaps by its inhibition of choline transport (Birks and MacIntosh, 1957; Schueler, 1960; Gardiner, 1961; MacIntosh, 1963). However, the results obtained should be interpreted with caution since HC-3 can inhibit ChE activity (Long, 1963) and can produce a "curare-like" action on the neuromuscular junction (Schueler, 1960). Evidence that HC-3 enters the brain after its systemic injection has been derived from its effects: (1) on central respiratory mechanisms (Borison, 1961; Metz, 1962); (2) somato-sensory evoked potentials recorded in the cuneate nucleus (Frazier and Boyarsky, 1964, 1967); and (3) on the release of ACh from the cerebral cortex (Szerb *et al.*, 1970). In "acute" experiments with dogs, intra-ventricularly-injected HC-3 (0·01–5 mg) caused highly-reproducible amygdaloid spiking and blocked hippocampal theta-wave activity, while not affecting neocortical activation (Domino, 1966; Domino *et al.*, 1967, 1968). However, the EEG effects caused by HC-3 varied with respect to the dose administered and were not consistent with those obtained with intravenous injections (Dren and Domino, 1968). The significant decreases in the ACh contents of amygdala, hippocampus, caudate nucleus, reticular formation and medial thalamus which were produced 4 h after administration of HC-3 (sometimes in the order of 50%, with 0·5 or 5 mg) led Dren and Domino (1968) to suggest that the EEG effects might be related to these changes. This idea was supported by the finding that exogenously-administered choline caused some reversal of the HC-3 effects (Domino *et al.*, 1967). Perhaps the most interesting aspect of these studies was the apparent "dissociation" which existed between neocortical- and limbic-activating mechanisms. This was shown not only with HC-3 but also when nicotine was used following pre-treatment with atropine. The latter results supported the previous finding of Torii and Wikler (1965) that atropine caused a "dissociation" between neocortical- and limbic-activation elicited by electrical stimulation of the reticular formation or posterior hypothalamus.

Is this "dissociation" due to the presence of distinctly different pathways? Studies of the effects of nicotine and arecoline on neocortical- and limbic-activation were aimed at answering this question. Kawamura and Domino (1969) showed, in cats transected at the caudal midbrain level, that nicotine (20–40 μg/kg, i.v.) activated both the neocortical and limbic (hippocampal) EEG by mechanisms which could be blocked by atropine, and that bilateral lesions of the MRF blocked nicotine (doses up to 100 $\mu$g/kg, i.v.)-induced activation of the forebrain EEG. In cats transected at the rostral midbrain region, nicotine (in doses up to 100 $\mu$g/kg) did not cause EEG activation while arecoline (20–40 $\mu$g/kg, i.v.) induced dissociation of the EEG between hippocampus and neocortex. It was concluded that nicotine caused activation of the rostral forebrain by an action primarily on the MRF, but that arecoline acted both rostral to the midbrain and on the MRF. It seems evident that the MRF is responsible for activating the neocortex while the hypothalamus activates predominantly the limbic system (see also Kawamura *et al.*, 1961; Kawamura and Domino, 1968). This seems interesting in that the hippocampus exerts a greater blocking effect than other areas of the cortex on conduction in the brainstem reticular formation (Adey *et al.*, 1957). From the above findings, it seems possible that cholinergic mechanisms may play a role in higher functions of the neocortex and hippocampus (i.e. motivation, learning and memory).

### 2.3 "Dissociation" of EEG and Behaviour

In the above section an apparent "dissociation" between two mechanisms of EEG activation has been discussed. These mechanisms must be related to the general behaviour of animals, and therefore it should be possible to dissociate gross behaviours from the EEG. Cholinergic agonists and antagonists can also be used for this purpose (e.g. Wikler, 1952; Bradley and Elkes, 1953, 1957; Bradley and Nicholson, 1962; see Longo, 1966). Treatment of animals with atropine can cause EEG patterns characteristic of "sleep" (high amplitude, slow-waves), but these patterns may or may not be reflected in behavioural sleep; i.e. animals may remain lively or drowsy (Wikler, 1952; Bradley, 1968; Bradley and Elkes, 1953, 1957). Therefore, atropine appears to disrupt the usual association between wakefulness and desynchronized EEG activity. This dissociation of EEG and behaviour, based on the action of atropine (Wikler, 1952), may be explained by the findings that mechanisms controlling sleep are located in the brain stem (see e.g. Jouvet, 1967), an area in which cholinoceptive elements do not have clear-cut muscarinic properties. Therefore, these mechanisms would not be blocked fully by atropine. Injections of eserine, and other anti-ChE agents, produce desynchronized EEG patterns which usually characterize behavioural arousal, but with eserine (as with atropine) animals may be either lively or drowsy (Bradley and Elkes, 1957; Monnier, 1959). The explanation of this dissociation of EEG and behaviour is complicated by the findings that certain cholinergic pathways may be involved in the induction of sleep (e.g. Hernández-Peón *et al.*,1963a, b).

Other studies have indicated that a dissociation between the EEG and ACh release can be caused by atropine and anti-ChE agents in "acute" cat preparations (e.g. Celesia and Jasper, 1966; see Chapter 6; Figs 6.1 and 6.2). In recent studies performed with freely-moving cats, Beani *et al.*, (1968) have shown that EEG changes, ACh release, and behaviour do not appear to be correlated with one another following the injection of atropine, and Jasper and Tessier (1971) found ACh release to be correlated to a greater extent with EEG activity than with behavioural responsiveness. The dissociation between EEG and behaviour may well have some functional significance, but at present this remains obscure.

## 2.4 Specific Sensory Systems

Recent results concerning the origin of the ACh released from the cerebral cortex by stimulation of visual and auditory pathways have led to two schools of thought: (1) that ACh release occurs mainly from the receiving areas of the cortex which are specific to the modality being stimulated and to a lesser extent by activation of the arousal mechanism (Collier and Mitchell, 1966, 1967; Hemsworth and Mitchell, 1969); (2) that the release of ACh from the cortex by both specific sensory and non-specific stimulation is due to activation of the reticulo-cortical arousal mechanism (Phillis, 1968a; Bartolini *et al.*, 1972; see Chapter 6). The

TABLE 2. Acetylcholine content of lateral geniculate bodies (LGB) and superior colliculus (SC)[a]. Reproduced with permission from Deffenu *et al.*, (1967).

| Conditions | No. | LGB Wt. (mg) | LGB ACh ($\mu$g/g) | No. | SC Wt. (mg) | SC ACh ($\mu$g/g) |
|---|---|---|---|---|---|---|
| Midpont. pretrig. transect. (contr.) | 4 | $67 \pm 7.5$ | $3.34 \pm 0.42$[b] | 4 | $108 \pm 10.4$ | $4.50 \pm 0.62$[c] |
| Midpont. pretrig. transect. + vis. deafferent. After 3 h | 7 | $59 \pm 7.5$ | $7.14 \pm 0.69$[b] | 6 | $113 \pm 3.9$ | $5.17 \pm 0.69$[c] |
| After 3 h and DOPA | 4 | $56 \pm 2.7$ | $3.82 \pm 0.45$[b] | 4 | $94 \pm 9.0$ | $3.44 \pm 0.71$[c] |
| "Cerveau isolé" | 2 | $50 \pm 6.4$ | $7.76 \pm 1.29$[b] | 1 | 95 | $5.13$[c] |

[a] All values $\pm$ S.E.M.
[b] The significance was determined by the analysis of variance; differences between these values are significant at $p < 0.01$.
[c] No significant differences were found between the weights and the ACh contents of SC.

writer has attempted to resolve this discrepancy (see §2.1). Since specific sensory pathways appear to have collaterals projecting to the arousal system, their stimulation could contribute to the diffuse release of ACh which is caused by reticulo-cortical activation (see Figs 2.1, 2.2 and 2.3). While electrical stimulation of the lateral or medial geniculate bodies is grossly unphysiological and could be expected to activate the arousal mechanism artifactually, photic (light flashes) or auditory (clicks) stimulation would not be expected to do this. Since a large portion of the ACh present in the lateral geniculate body (LGB) of the cat may be related to fibres originating in the reticular formation (Deffenu *et al.*,

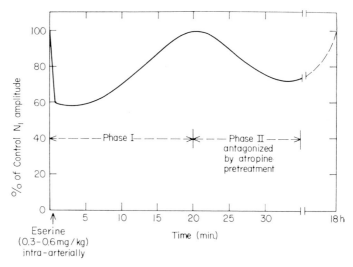

FIG. 2.14. Inhibition of auditory nerve action potentials by eserine (physostigmine) in the cat. Auditory nerve action potentials, designated as $N_1$ when recorded from the round window of the inner ear, were obtained in response to clicks. Intra-arterial injections of eserine (0·3–0·6 mg/kg) produced, in most animals, an inhibition (*Phase I*) and a secondary inhibition (*Phase II*) of slow onset and long duration. The Phase II inhibition could be prevented by pretreatment with atropine. Note that olivo-cochlear bundle-induced inhibition has also been shown to inhibit $N_1$ (e.g. Besmedt, 1962; Fex, 1962). Reproduced with permission from Amaro *et al.*, (1966).

1966, 1967), some portion of visual stimulation may reach the cortex by way of the arousal pathway. With regard to the visual pathway itself, the LGB and superior colliculus of the cat contain very high concentrations of ACh (Widen and Ajmone-Marsan, 1960; Deffenu *et al.*, 1966, 1967) and considerable ChAc activity (Hebb and Silver, 1956). Deffenu *et al.*, (1967) showed that at 3 h after visual de-afferentation of cats, ACh content was markedly increased in LGB and increased to some extent in the superior colliculus (Table 2). Intravenous injection of D

L-DOPA (30 mg/kg) caused activation of the cortex and prevented the change in ACh content of the LGB (Table (2)). David *et al.*, (1963) concluded from studies with iontophoretic methods that at least one mechanism in the LGB is cholinergic. In a recent study, Stevens (1973) showed that light responses in cells of the frog optic tectum were reduced by topically applied ACh or nicotine, and he concluded that visual processing in tectal cells might be mediated by inhibitory systems which contain nicotinic cholinergic synapses. A cholinergic role in vision also seems evident from other studies (see Phillis, 1970, 1971).

With regard to the auditory system, physiological and pharmacological studies on olivo-cochlear inhibition have revealed that this system

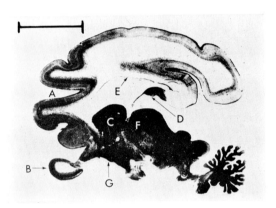

Fig. 2.15. AChE activity in a parasagittal section of a kitten's brain. (A) Cruciate sulcus; (B) olfactory bulb; (C) caudate nucleus; (D) hippocampus; (E) "subcallosal band"; (F) thalmus; (G) olfactory tubercle. Thiocholine method. Scale: 10 mm. Reproduced with permission from Krnjević and Silver (1965).

may operate by a cholinergic mechanism (e.g. Gisselson, 1952; Amaro *et al.*, 1966; Daigneault and Brown, 1966; Fex, 1968; Guth and Amaro, 1969; Bobbin and Konishi, 1971; see Fig. 2.14). It has been well established that within the cochlea of the inner ear only the terminals of the olivo-cochlear bundle (OCB) stain for AChE (Churchill *et al.*, 1956; Vinnikov and Titova, 1958; Schuknecht *et al.*, 1959; Hilding and Wersall, 1962; Shute and Lewis, 1965; Rossi and Cortesina, 1965), and that AChE is clearly associated with crossed OCB nerve endings in the cochlea (Rossi and Cortesina, 1966; see also Schuknecht, 1958). Also, ACh may be released from the OCB when it is stimulated (Norris *et al.*, 1972). Further support for the contention that olivo-cochlear transmission is cholinergic derives from studies which showed that section and degeneration of crossed and uncrossed OCB reduced significantly the ChAc activity in cranial nerve VIII (auditory nerve) and in the membranous cochlea (Jasser and Guth, 1973). Hence, there appears to be good evidence in support of an acoustic role for the central cholinergic system (see also Phillis, 1970, 1971).

Since cholinergic synapses may exist in the mammalian olfactory bulb (Von Baumgarten *et al.*, 1963; Salmoiraghi *et al.*, 1964) and medial geniculate nucleus (see refs in Phillis, 1970), and since rhinencephalic structures are rich in ACh, ChAc and AChE (see e.g. Krnjević and Silver, 1965; Hebb and Morrris, 1969; Hebb and Silver, 1970; Fig. 2.15), it seems possible that cholinergic mechanisms may also play a significant role in olfaction. Studies which have shown that ACh can be released from various brain areas by peripheral nerve stimulation indicate that mechanisms conveying proprioceptive sense and discriminative touch to higher levels of the neuraxis may have cholinergic components or may cause activation of the cholinergic arousal mechanism (see Figs 2.1, 2.2 and 2.3 and Chapter 6).

### 2.5 The Link Between Cholinergic and Adrenergic Arousal

Mechanisms involved in "arousal", "sleep-wakefulness" and the "dissociation of EEG and behaviour" are obviously too complex to be explained simply in terms of central cholinergic systems. In terms of chemical transmitter theory, these mechanisms will not be explained until the central roles of other possible transmitter systems (e.g. those involving glutamate and GABA) are more clearly defined. Evidence that "links" may exist between central cholinergic, adrenergic, and amino acid mechanisms is really just emerging, although the early "alternation hypothesis" of Feldberg and Vogt (1948) certainly predicted that such evidence would be required to explain the transmitter processes underlying complex physiological and behavioural phenomena. Jouvet (1969) has hypothesized that nor-adrenaline (NA), dopamine (DA), and serotonin (5-HT) might be involved in the sleep-wakefulness cycle, and recently Jasper and Koyama (1969) have suggested that glutamate and some other "active" amino acids might play significant roles in mediating arousal. In this section, evidence which supports the existence of an interplay between cholinergic and adrenergic mechanisms in the regulation of arousal will be briefly discussed.

Grossman (1968) showed that reversible behavioural changes could be produced by direct application of cholinergic and adrenergic substances to restricted portions of the MRF of freely-moving rats. Cholinergic drugs increased markedly the animal's reactivity to supra-threshold stimuli while NA caused depressant effects. Hence, both cholinergic and adrenergic mechanisms seemed to be involved in the regulation of an animal's responsiveness to sensory input (i.e. in its level of arousal). In developmental studies along this line, Fibiger *et al.*, (1970) showed that pilocarpine decreased amphetamine-induced psychomotor excitation in 20–25-day-old rats, but not in younger rats. It was concluded that an adrenergic arousal system was perhaps present at very early ages, but that at approximately 20 days of age a cholinergic inhibitory system predominated. Reviews of the literature have led to the idea that the biochemical substrates for behavioural arousal are adrenergic (Carlton, 1963; Schildkraut and Kety, 1967), and it has been suggested that the effects of cholinergic stimulation oppose the effects of adrenergic stimulation (e.g. Pfeiffer and Jenny, 1957). Zetler (1968) showed that behavioural inhibition can be produced by several centrally-acting cholinergic agonists (see also Carlton, 1963, 1969, and Chapter 5). However, most of the studies involved in these analyses were made using systemic injections.

Perhaps, the best evidence, though indirect, for the existence of a cholinergic-adrenergic link in the arousal mechanism has been obtained from studies of the effects of amphetamines on central cholinergic mechanisms. It is well known that amphetamines promote a release of catecholamines from adrenergic nerve endings (e.g. Randrup and Munkvad, 1966; Hanson, 1967; Boakes *et al.*, 1971). Also, in earlier studies it was shown that systemic injections of amphetamines antagonized a number of the behavioural effects caused by atropine and scopolamine (*1*-hyoscine) in rats, rabbits, dogs and monkeys (White and Daigneault, 1959; White *et al.*, 1961; Pazzagli and Pepeu, 1964). Studies on the central release of ACh have provided further evidence for this proposed adrenergic-cholinergic link in that injected amphetamines increase ACh release from the cerebral cortex (Pepeu and Bartolini, 1967, 1968; Hemsworth and Neal, 1968; Bartolini and Pepeu, 1970). From the results obtained with midbrain-transected cats, Pepeu and Bartolini (1968) suggested that amphetamine increased cortical ACh release by activating catecholaminergic nerve terminals which synapse on cholinergic neurones in rostral brain structures (see Fig. 6.22). Histochemical studies of the distribution of catecholamines in the CNS have supported the hypothesis that catecholamines may serve transmitter roles in behavioural arousal (e.g. Andén *et al.*, 1966; Fuxe and Hanson, 1967).

It had been postulated that the increase in cortical ACh release and the EEG activation caused by amphetamine administration depended on having part of the reticular formation intact (Deffenu *et al.*, 1970; see also Bradley and Elkes, 1953; Hiebel *et al.*, 1954), but recently Nistri *et al.*, (1972) have shown, in cats, that the effect of the amphetamine on cortical ACh release might not be mediated by its action on the reticular formation. Amphetamine-induced increases in ACh release have also been effectively prevented by administration of chlorpromazine (Pepeu and Bartolini, 1968; Nistri *et al.*, 1972) or propranolol

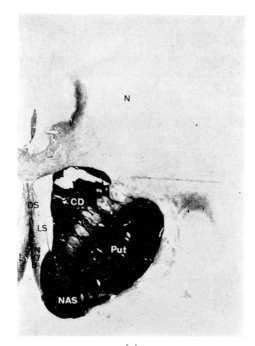

(a)

(b)

FIG. 2.16 (a) and (b). Frontal sections of *Cebus* monkey brain showing AChE activity. Note the intensely-stained nucleus accumbens septi in (a), and the septal nuclei and intensely-stained basal ganglia in (b). *CD*, Caudate nucleus; *DS*, dorsal septal nucleus; *LS*, lateral septal nucleus; *N*, neocortex; *NAS*, nucleus accumbens septi; *NDB*, nucleus of diagonal band of Broca; *Put*, putamen. Thiocholine method (×5). Reproduced with permission from Girgis (1973).

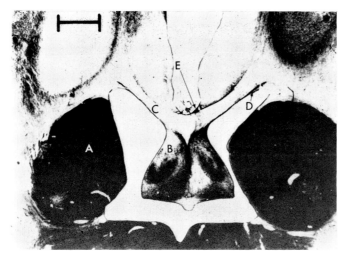

FIG. 2.17. Horizontal section of kitten's forebrain showing AChE activity. Note intensely-stained caudate nuclei and strong staining in the septum. The latter is directly continuous with the "subcallosal band" and is linked by "perforating fibres" with the induseum griseum and other parts of the supracallosal formation. *A*, Caudate nucleus; *B*, septum; *C*, corpus callosum; *D*, "subcallosal band"; *E*, induseum griseum. Thiocholine method. Scale: 2·0 mm. Reproduced with permission from Krnjević and Silver (1965).

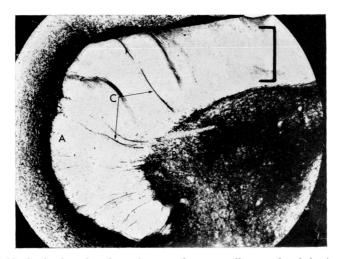

FIG. 2.18. Sagittal section through genu of corpus callosum of cat's brain showing AChE activity. The strongly stained medial septal nucleus is linked with the supracallosal formation by "perforating fibres". *A*, Genu; *B*, septum; *C*, "perforating fibres". Thiocholine method. Scale: 1·0 mm. Reproduced with permission from Krnjević and Silver (1965).

(Bartolini and Pepeu, 1970), or by destruction of a large portion of the diencephalon (Deffenu *et al.*, 1970). Nistri *et al.*, (1972) have suggested that amphetamine might increase cortical ACh output by causing a release of catecholamines which could then activate a cholinergic pathway which may either originate in, or traverse, the septum and which projects to the cerebral cortex. In these studies, destruction of the septal area prevented amphetamine-induced increases in cortical ACh release. It seems likely that an anatomical locus linking adrenergic and cholinergic mechanisms of arousal may exist in the septal area. It has been shown both histochemically and physiologically that the septum is rich in both cholinergic and adrenergic elements (see e.g. Krnjević and Silver, 1965; Lewis and Shute, 1967; Lewis *et al.*, 1967; Szerb, 1967; Fuxe *et al.*, 1969; Pepeu *et al.*, 1971; King and Jewett, 1971; Girgis, 1973; Figs 2.16–2.18), and that it is involved in emotion and in motivated behaviours (see below and Chapter 5).

*Chapter 3*

# Cholinergic Roles in Motor Systems

### 3.1 Posture and Reflexes

Since much evidence has indicated that spinal motoneurones are cholinergic (see e.g. reviews by Eccles, 1964; Phillis, 1970; Figs 3.1 and 3.2, and Kása *et al.*, 1970a, b), there seems to be little doubt that central cholinergic systems are associated with the reflex regulation of movement and with postural mechanisms. However, it must be understood that postural mechanisms are complex and that their explanation requires discussion of reticulo-cortical, extrapyramidal and cerebellar mechanisms as well as spinal reflex activities. In this section, an effort will be made to define the cholinergic nature of some spinal mechanisms which seem to be involved in reflexes and posture.

It has been long known that injections of nicotine into the spinal blood supply can inhibit motoneuronal reflex discharges (e.g. Schweitzer and Wright, 1938; Bülbring and Burn, 1941; Curtis *et al.*, 1957), but similar injections of ACh do not cause consistent reflex inhibition (Curtis *et al.*, 1957). However, spinal reflexes have been depressed rather reliably by intra-thecal injections of ACh or neostigmine in man, though some excitatory actions were also evident (Kremer, 1942). It had been suggested that systemic injections of ACh can produce excitation of spinal motoneurones (see Feldberg, 1945, 1950), but more recent iontophoretic studies have indicated that these cells are very insensitive to ACh (Curtis *et al.*, 1961).

Antidromic stimulation of a given muscle nerve is known to produce both inhibition and facilitation of monosynaptic reflex activity in other muscle nerves (Renshaw, 1941), and both antidromic and orthodromic stimulation of motoneurones can activate recurrent collateral fibres which can lead to the inhibition or facilitation of neighbouring motoneurones (e.g. Eccles *et al.*, 1954; Wilson, 1959). It has been suggested that the pathways for both "recurrent inhibition" and "recurrent facilitation" (a "disinhibitory phenomenon", perhaps occurring by

33

the release of "tonic" inhibition of motoneurones) contain a cholinergic synapse (Wilson, 1959; Wilson *et al.*, 1960; Wilson and Burgess, 1962). Since Renshaw cells appear to be the only spinal neurones which are consistently excited by ACh, it has been maintained that these cells become activated by impulses in recurrent collaterals of motoneurones (Eccles *et al.*, 1954, 1956; Granit *et al.*, 1957; Curtis *et al.*, 1957; Curtis

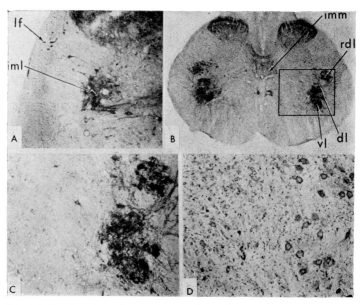

Fig. 3.1. (*A*), Section through sacral part of rat spinal cord showing AChE activity in the intermediolateral column (*iml*) and in cells of the lateral white funiculus (*lf*), ×90. (*B*) Section through spinal cord at level of last lumbar segment showing AChE activity in the three lateral sub-column's (*rdl*, *dl* and *vl*) and in the intermediomedial column (*imm*). ×30. (*C*), Enlargement of caged area of *B*, showing AChE activity in the ventral horn (×90). Modified thiocholine method for *A*, *B* and *C*. *D*, Section through the AChE-negative area of the ventral horn stained with cresyl violet showing numerous neurones which were usually smaller than motoneurones. Reproduced with permission from Navaratnam and Lewis (1970).

and Eccles, 1958a, b; Granit and Rutledge, 1960; Granit *et al.*, 1960, 1961; Wilson *et al.*, 1960). The recurrent inhibition caused by Renshaw cell activation of motoneurones (see monograph by Eccles, 1969; Fig. 3.2) seems to be more selective to "tonically-active" motoneurones which are likely to be associated with postural mechanisms (Granit *et al.*, 1957, 1960, 1961; see monograph by Granit, 1970).

Although the axon collateral-Renshaw cell synapse is considered to be one of the best examples of a cholinergic synapse in the CNS, the positive identification of Renshaw cells (or of this synapse) has not been anatomically established (Scheibel and Scheibel, 1966; Erulkar *et al.*, 1968). This has led to an alternative explanation of recurrent inhibition. Weight (1968) believes that motoneuronal axon collaterals may synapse directly with motoneurones, and therefore that Renshaw cells may not be necessary for recurrent inhibition. This notion derives support from

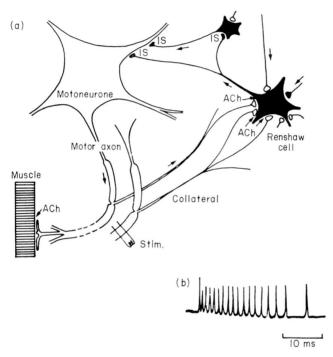

FIG. 3.2. (a), Diagram of the inhibitory pathways to motoneurones by their axon collaterals and Renshaw cells. (b), Extracellular recording of Renshaw cell being excited by an antidromic volley in the motor fibres of lateral gastrocnemius muscle. Inhibitory cells are in *black*; *IS* = inhibitory synapse. Reproduced with permission from Eccles (1969).

the studies of Erulkar *et al.*, (1968) which indicated that stained "Renshaw elements" localized on motoneuronal surfaces resembled the "boutons termineaux" of motoneurones rather than interneuronal perikarya. However, in order for Weight's theory to hold, the ACh released by motoneuronal axon collaterals should cause direct inhibition of motoneurones. This would not be in accord with the finding of Curtis *et al.* (1961) that iontophoretically-applied ACh has no action on spinal motoneurones. If it is shown that another substance which can inhibit motoneuronal firing is liberated by axon collaterals, then Weight's

theory might be valid. In a recent review by Willis (1971) it was concluded that Renshaw cells are likely to exist and that there are no
good reasons to believe that these are "boutons termineaux" of motoneurones or motoneuronal dendritic processes.

### 3.2 Tremors and Catalepsy: Extrapyramidal System

Much evidence has accumulated to support a role for cholinergic
mechanisms in extrapyramidal motor functions, which are known to be
associated with the involuntary control of movement and with posture.
Perturbations of the extrapyramidal system with centrally-active cholinergic agents cause Parkinsonian-like tremors, other dyskinesias, catalepsy, "circling" behaviours, and related disturbances (e.g. Mennear,
1965; Timsit, 1966; Arnfred and Randrup, 1968; Costall *et al.*, 1972).
The nuclei which comprise the extrapyramidal system (globus pallidus,
caudate nucleus, putamen, substantia nigra) contain large amounts of
ACh, AChE and ChAc (see e.g. Gerebtzoff, 1959; Krnjević and Silver,
1965; Lewis and Shute, 1967; Fahn and Coté, 1968; Girgis, 1973; Figs
2.5, 2.15–2.18, 3.5–3.7). The globus pallidus also contains higher concentrations of iron (Spatz, 1922) and Vitamin $B_2$ (riboflavine) (Diezel
and Taubert, 1954) than other brain structures. Intense, interest in the
globus pallidus has been stimulated by the demonstration by Spiegel *et
al.*, (1947) that its disjunction diminishes or abolishes Parkinsonian tremor
in humans. A significant role for the globus pallidus in rest tremor (RT)
has been supported further by the recent findings that: (1) destruction
of this structure decreased contralateral RT in rats, and directly-
injected oxotremorine induced RT (Blažević *et al.*, 1965; (2) infusion of
ACh into this structure produced RT (Ruždik and Stern, 1966); (3)
direct injections of hemicholinium-3 (HC-3), or other anticholinergic
agents, into this structure prevented RT (Nashold, 1959; Ruždik, 1965).
It has been shown further that administration of both tremorine (Pepeu,
1963; Holmstedt *et al.*, 1963) and its active metabolite, oxotremorine
(Holmstedt and Lundgren, 1966), cause increases in the total ACh
content of brain. The caudate nucleus has also been under intensive
investigation since its content of DA is decreased in patients afflicted
with Parkinsonism (Ehringer and Hornykiewics, 1960; Hornykiewics,
1960). Further evidence for the involvement of cholinergic mechanisms
in Parkinsonism derives from the clinical effectiveness of cholinergic
antagonists (e.g. atropine) in relieving Parkinsonian tremor (e.g. Friedman and Everett, 1964) and from recent results which have indicated
that a balance between the levels of ACh and DA in extrapyramidal
structures may be involved in the "tremor-regulating" mechanism (e.g.
Barbeau, 1962; Schelkunov, 1967; Connor *et al.*, 1967; Dill *et al.*, 1968;
Klawans, 1968; Larochelle *et al.*, 1971). An interrelationship of ACh

and DA in the extrapyramidal system may also be involved in catalepsy (e.g. Timsit, 1966; Morpurgo and Theobald, 1964; Costall and Olley, 1971a; Larochelle *et al.*, 1971) and in "circling" behaviours (e.g. Stevens *et al.*, 1961; Hull *et al.*, 1967; Ungerstedt *et al.*, 1969; Costall *et al.*, 1972; Figs 3.3, 3.15 and 3.16). Recent studies have indicated that the induction of catalepsy by administration of neuroleptic agents[1] depends upon

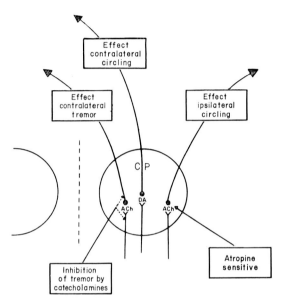

Fig. 3.3. Diagram illustrating the possible involvement of cholinergic (ACh) and dopaminergic (DA) systems in the candate-putamen (CP) with tremor and circling behaviours. Reproduced with permission from Costall *et al.*, (1972).

dopaminergic innervation of both mesolimbic and extrapyramidal systems (Andén *et al.*, 1970; Andén, 1972; Costall and Naylor, 1973).

Other results have indicated that the ACh contents of certain central structures are increased during RT (Bordeleau, 1961), and that the increases in brain ACh content caused by anti-ChE agents occur concomitantly with RT (Erdmann and Teutloff, 1963). The muscarinic agents, tremorine and oxotremorine, have been studied most extensively with regard to extrapyramidal mechanisms. These agents produce, by

---

[1] Neuroleptic agents (e.g. phenothiazine and butyrophenone tranquilizers) perhaps act by increasing the "turnover" of DA. This may occur by "feedback activation" of DA release, which could be caused by blockade of post-synaptic DA receptors by the neuroleptic agent (see Andén *et al.*, 1970).

their actions on the basal ganglia, behavioural symptoms in experimental animals which resemble those of Parkinsonism (Everett, 1956, 1961; Cho *et al.*, 1961, 1962), while increasing cerebral ACh content (see above). Since tremorine must be metabolized to oxotremorine in order to produce tremors (Cho *et al.*, 1961), the latter drug has been most widely employed in the more recent studies; similar effects are produced by either drug. At present, it is not known with certainty whether the increase in brain ACh content caused by these agents is strictly localized to the extra-pyramidal system, or whether this change is causally related to the tremor produced. However, in this connection, Bartolini *et al.*, (1970) showed that within a few minutes after systemic injection of oxotremorine (1 mg/kg) into cats, tremor occurred and that ACh levels were increased in diencephalon and upper midbrain. In other studies, injections of tremorine (5 mg/kg) into dogs produced only slight increases in the ACh contents of motor cortex and caudate nucleus, while decreasing significantly the ACh content of the globus pallidus (Hadžović *et al.*, 1966). It has been shown further that oxotremorine is most effective at increasing the ACh content of homogenates prepared from brain regions containing caudate nucleus, globus pallidus and substantia nigra (Lundgren and Malmburg, 1968). The above studies correlate well with those of Cox and Potkonjak (1969) who found that direct injections of tremorine into these same nuclei elicited tremor in rats (see also Blažević *et al.*, 1965). Since the quaternary analogue of oxotremorine (N-methyloxotremorine), which exerts pronounced peripheral parasympathomimetic effects with little central action, caused only a minimal elevation of cerebral ACh and no centrally-mediated behavioural response, and since N-methyl-atropine did not inhibit the oxotremorine-induced increase in brain ACh, it seems likely that the oxotremorine-induced increases in brain ACh content occurred by a direct central action (see Campbell *et al.*, 1970).

Other studies have led to the view that oxotremorine may not act exclusively by its interaction with central cholinergic mechanisms. Hadžović *et al.*, (1965) found that injections of tremorine caused significant decreases in both the iron and copper contents of rat brain, and Stern *et al.*, (1966) showed that tremorine caused a reduction of iron in corpus striatum but not in cerebral cortex or white matter of rabbit brain (see also Stern *et al.*, 1969; Table 3). In Table 3, it is shown further that at about 1 h after the initial decrease in iron content of rat brain mitochondria, there occurred an increase. By killing rats 30 min. after injection of oxotremorine, it was shown that non-haem iron was not affected by the drug (Table 4). Earlier experiments by Emerson and Tischler (1944) had indicated that intravenously-administered iso-riboflavine (a riboflavine antagonist) enhanced the tremor produced by oxotremorine, an effect which was opposite to that produced by ribo-flavine, itself. Stern and Hasanagić (1967) showed further that oxotre-morine decreases total brain flavines (see also Stern *et al.*, 1969; Table 3).

TABLE 3. Changes of total iron and flavines in rat brain corpora striata after oxotremorine (0·25 mg/kg, i.v.). Reproduced with permission from Stern *et al.* (1969).

| Time after injection (min.) | Total iron Per cent of control values (number of animals) | Total flavines Per cent of control values (number of animals) |
|---|---|---|
| 15 | 77·6[a](6) | 102·9 (6) |
| 30 | 76·4[a](8) | 98·0 (6) |
| 60 | 101·7 (7) | 96·1 (7) |
| 90 | 121·3[a](7) | 73·0[a](7) |
| 120 | 142·8[a](7) | 65·5[a](6) |

[a] Differences between these values and controls were statistically significant at the $p < 0.005$ level (*t*-test). Control values were obtained from nine animals.

Note that oxotremorine treatment exerted a biphasic effect on the iron content of mito-chondria while causing a significant decrease in flavine content at about 90 minutes.

Hence, the RT produced by oxotremorine may be caused by its inhibi-tion of riboflavine action as well as by its action of increasing cerebral ACh content (see Stern, 1967). These findings have indicated that the increase in cerebral ACh caused by oxotremorine, or the tremor which it induces (or RT, itself), may occur secondarily to changes produced in cytochrome systems and/or in enzyme systems involved in cerebral energy metabolism (see below). Another mechanism for explaining the central actions of tremorine (oxotremorine) might be derived from its ability to stimulate ChAc activity *in vivo* (Ratković *et al.*, 1965).

Experiments with tremorine have added still another dimension to the possible origin of Parkinsonian-like RT. It is well known that the globus pallidus is hyperactive in Parkinsonian patients (Pakkenberg, 1963), presumably due to an "overriding" effect of cholinergic excitation on dopaminergic inhibition, and it has been postulated that the globus pallidus may be a "pacemaker" for RT (Lamarre and Cordeau, 1963). Also, the intensity of tremor produced by injections of tremorine in rats is decreased by bilateral destruction of the globus pallidus (Blažević *et al.*, 1965). It seems possible, therefore, that hyperactivity of the globus pallidus may serve to free spinal motoneurones from supra-spinal influences. However, in the studies of Chalmers and Yim (1963), section of the spinal cord in rats and dogs did not relieve the tremor produced by tremorine, and hence, this tremor could have been caused by "automatism" of ventral horn cells. Further evidence that tremorine exerts a direct action on ventral horn cells has been reported (Stern, 1964; Bošković *et al.*, 1964; Blažević *et al.*, 1967). In this connection, the

TABLE 4. Changes in total and non-haem iron in mitochondria of rat corpora striata 30 min after oxotremorine (0·25 mg/kg, i.v.). Reproduced with permission from Stern *et al.*, (1969).

| | Iron $\mu$g/mg (wet) | |
|---|---|---|
| | Total | Non-heme |
| Control | 79·7 ± 8·8 (8)[a] | 14·8 ± 3·9 (8)[a] |
| Experimental | 60·9 ± 3·7 (8)[a] | 13·8 ± 4·4 (8)[a] |
| Relative change (%) of control | −23·5 | n.s.[b] |

[a] Numbers of determinations are given in parentheses.
[b] "n.s." means statistically non-significant at the 0·05 level (*t*-test).

increases in ChAc activity caused by tremorine (Ratković *et al.*, 1965) could have caused an accumulation of ACh in spinal motoneurones and/or an increase in their release of ACh (Stern and Gašparović, 1962; Ratković *et al.*, 1965) which could have been related to the changes in excitability which were observed.

Further evidence supporting a relationship between cholinergic mechanisms and tremor has been provided by studies in which other cholinomimetic or cholinolytic agents have been applied directly to extrapyramidal structures. Marked species differences exist in the sensitivity of extrapyramidal structures to directly-applied ACh or other cholinergic agents. This was predictable since stimulation or destruction of the caudate nucleus in the rat did not affect RT (Whittier and Orr, 1962), while in man and other mammals RT depends heavily on the caudate nucleus. However, infusion of ACh into the globus pallidus in rats does cause RT which can be reduced by ablating this structure or by applying cholinolytic agents such HC-3 (Ruždić, 1965). Tremors can also be produced by injecting carbachol directly into the head of the caudate nucleus of the conscious cat, and this response is quite specific for this structure (Connor *et al.*, 1966a; Lalley *et al.*, 1970; Table 5).

TABLE 5. Tremor characteristics produced by intra-caudate injection of carbachol, eserine, di-isopropyl-fluorophosphate (DFP), or echothiophate (ECHO)[a]. Reproduced with permission from Lalley *et al.*, (1970).

| Cholinergic agents and tremor activity Tremorigenic parameters | Pharmacologic Carbachol[b] | Endogenous: Anticholinesterases | | |
|---|---|---|---|---|
| | | Eserine (Reversible) | DFP | ECHO Irreversible) |
| Dose ($\mu$g) | 7 (5–8) | 150 (100–200) | 32 (25–60) | 23 (15–30) |
| Latency (min) | 14 (9–21) | 32 (13–40) | 7 (1–18) | 13 (7–35) |
| Maximal tremor characteristics: | | | | |
| Onset of peak effect (min) | 34 (20–50) | 56 (30–118) | 56 (35–71) | 52 (40–76) |
| Duration of maximal tremor (min) | 92 (70–100) | 112 (60–300) | 150[c] (90–180) | 90[c] (66–118) |
| Amplitude (graded intensity) | (++) | (++) | (+) | (+) |
| Bursts/min | 21 (16–28) | 19 (10–27) | 25 (18–33) | 26 (21–30) |
| Tremor frequency (cycles/sec) | 20 (16–23) | 22 (18–25) | 21 (18–25) | 20 (15–25) |
| Tremor time (%) | 74 (66–83) | 49 (25–65) | 45 (24–60) | 48 (39–58) |
| Residual Tremor | (−) | (−) | (+) | (+) |

[a] Mean values (ranges in parentheses) for carbachol derived from 18 experiments; those for DFP, ECHO, and eserine derived from 8, 9 and 14 experiments, respectively.
[b] Values reported for carbachol are based on results which had been, in part, previously reported (Connor *et al.* (1966a)).
[c] Calculated during acute period of maximal tremor; residual tremor at reduced activity was recorded for weeks after a single injection of the irreversible anticholinesterases.

Using this same technique, Baker *et al.*, (1967a) found that the tremor elicited by cholinergic agents (e.g. carbachol) may be mediated by muscarinic receptors. Intra-caudate injections of anti-ChE agents also caused tremor (perhaps by promoting an accumulation of endogenous ACh), which was abolished by muscarinic blocking agents, catecholamines or ATP (Baker *et al.*, 1967a; Table 6). These results indicated

TABLE 6. Effects of intra-caudate injections of cholinergic antagonists on tremor induced by carbachol (or DFP). Reproduced with permission from Baker *et al.*, (1967a).

| Cholinergic antagonists and their principal receptor activities | Tremor antagonism | Dose[a] (μg) | Latency (min.) | Duration (min.) | Ratio: $\left[\dfrac{\text{Tremor antagonism}}{\text{Total experiments}}\right]$ |
|---|---|---|---|---|---|
| Muscarinic: | | | | | |
| Scopolamine | (+) | 25 (18–31) | 7 (3–9) | 190 (145–212) | 24/24 |
| Scopolamine (against DFP) | (+) | 58 (25–113) | 10 (2–30) | 115[b] | 8/10 |
| Benztropine | (+) | 100 (75–110) | 21 (19–24) | 76 (69–89) | 6/6 |
| Nicotinic: | | | | | |
| *Ganglionic blockers* | | | | | |
| Hexamethonium | (−) | —[c] | ⋯ | ⋯ | 0/6 |
| Nicotine (large doses) | (−) | —[c] | ⋯ | ⋯ | 0/9 |
| *Neuromuscular blockers* | | | | | |
| Dihydro-β-erythroidine | (−) | —[d] | ⋯ | ⋯ | 0/6 |
| *d*-Tubocurarine | (−) | —[d] | ⋯ | ⋯ | 0/6 |

Mean values (ranges in parentheses) were derived from experiments on at least 6 different cats.

[a] Mean dose completely abolishing tremor.

[b] Total duration was determined only in 2 experiments (2 cats); duration of antagonism in other 6 experiments was followed for a period of only 30 minutes.

[c] Failed to abolish tremor at cumulative doses to 300 μg.

[d] Failed to abolish tremor at cumulative doses to 100 μg.

that a link may exist between the actions of ACh and catecholamines (e.g. DA) with regard to caudate function (see below), and confirmed other findings in which muscarinic receptor mechanisms were implicated in central cholinergic function (see e.g. Chapter 6, and reviews by Eccles, 1964; Krnjević, 1964, 1965a; Curtis and Crawford, 1969; Phillis, 1970). Intra-caudate injections of anti-ChE agents have also provided evidence which led to the suggestion that an elevation of ACh might cause a release of DA in this structure (Lalley *et al.*, 1970; Table 5). These results support the hypothesis that both ACh and DA are involved in the regulation of Parkinsonian-like tremor.

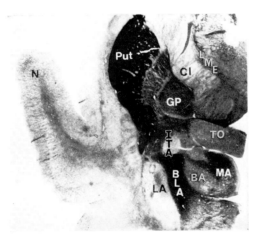

Fig. 3.4. Frontal section of *Cebus* monkey brain at the cranial end of the uncus showing AChE activity in some amygdaloid nuclei, in the basal ganglia and in some other structures. Note that the globus pallidus stains much less than the putamen. *BA*, accessory basal amygdaloid nucleus; *BLA*, basal amygdaloid nucleus; *Cl*, internal capsule; *GP*, globus pallidus; *ITA*, intercalculated mass of cells (amygdala); *LA*, lateral amygdaloid nucleus; *LME*, external medullary lamina of thalamus; *MA*, medial amygdaloid nucleus; *N*, neocortex; *Put*, putamen; *TO*, opic tract. Thiocholine method (×5). Reproduced with permission from Girgis (1973).

Another useful approach for the study of central cholinergic pathways in relation to tremorigenic mechanisms has been based on histochemical methods. It has been well established that high concentrations of ACh (MacIntosh, 1941) and high ChAc (Hebb and Silver, 1956; Fahn and Coté, 1968) and AChE activities are present in cells and nerve fibres of the internal capsule, globus pallidus, substantia nigra and related structures (e.g. Krnjević and Silver, 1965; Olivier *et al.*, 1970; Girgis, 1973; Figs 2.5, 2.15–2.17, 3.4–3.6) and that many striatal fibres terminate in b th divisions of the globus pallidus (Szabo, 1962; Nauta and

Mehler, 1966; Olivier *et al.*, 1970). It has been suggested on the basis of lesion studies and AChE staining that the pathways from the striatum to the globus pallidus and substantia nigra are rather exclusively cholinergic (Olivier *et al.*, 1970; see Figs 3.6 and 3.7). Since these workers found that unilateral lesions of the ventral midbrain tegmentum, which produced a complete cell loss in the ipsilateral substantia nigra, did not

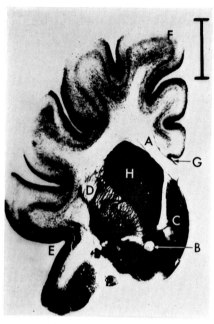

FIG. 3.5. Frontal section of cat's forebrain showing distribution of AChE activity. *A*, Corpus callosum; *B*, anterior commissure; *C*, septum; *D*, internal capsule; *E*, rhinal fissure; *F*, marginal gyrus; *G*, induseum griseum; *H*, caudate nucleus. Thiocholine method. Scale: 5 mm. Reproduced with permission from Krnjević and Silver (1965).

affect the AChE activity in fibres rostral to the lesion, it was concluded that these are descending striato-nigral (strionigral) fibres, a finding which is not in accord with the previous results of Shute and Lewis (1963) who concluded that these were nigro-striatal fibres. Other evidence has indicated that some of these cholinergic fibres may synapse with dopaminergic cells of the substantia nigra (Smelik and Ernst, 1966) and that some dopaminergic fibres of the substantia nigra project to the striatum (Andén *et al.*, 1964; Poirier and Sourkes, 1964, 1965). Since nigrostriatal lesions affect tyrosine hydroxylase, striatal dopamine (DA) synthesis might be regulated by a cholinergic mechanism (see Goldstein *et al.*, 1966; Poirier *et al.*, 1969; Olivier *et al.*, 1970). Strionigral

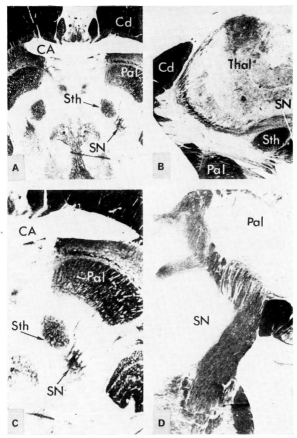

Fig. 3.6. (A) Horizontal section through upper brain stem of a normal monkey showing the distribution of cholinesterase in various structures. Note particularly the intensity of staining in the striatum, globus pallidus, subthalamic nucleus, substantia nigra and strionigral fibres. Thiocholine method (×3). (B) Sagittal section through upper brain stem showing cholinesterase activity in the caudate nucleus, globus pallidus, reticular nucleus of the thalamus, subthalamic nucleus, substantia nigra and strionigral fibres. Thiocholine method (×3). (C) Same as (A) at a higher magnification (×5) to illustrate more clearly the strionigral fibres and comb bundle. (D) Horizontal section through upper brain stem showing the appearance of structures stained for cells and myelin. Fast blue and basic fuchsin (×5). *CA*, anterior commissure; *Cd*, caudate nucleus; *Sth*, subthalamic nucleus; *SN*, substantia nigra; *Thal*, thalamus; *Pal*, globus pallidus. Reproduced with permission from Olivier *et al.*, (1970).

fibres, which are presumed to project to dopaminergic neurones of the substantia nigra, arc better developed in monkey than in cat (see Olivier *et al.*, 1970), and hence may be associated with Parkinsonism and other related disorders of man. The cholinesterasic strionigral fibres (Olivier

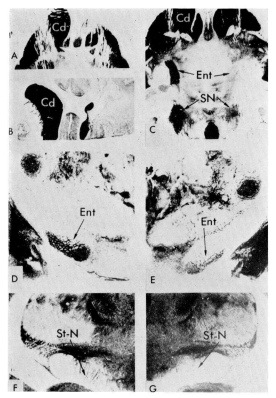

Fig. 3.7. Effects of lesions of the caudate nucleus on cholinesterase activity. (A) Horizontal section through the striatum showing unilateral lesion of the caudate nucleus in a cat that survived 78 days (×2·5). (B) Transverse section through the striatum showing a unilateral lesion of the caudate nucleus in a cat that survived 90 days (×2·5). (C) Horizontal section through the upper brain stem of the same animal as shown in (A); note the marked disappearance of cholinesterase activity in the entopeduncular nucleus and at the level of the rostral substantia nigra on the side of the lesion (×3). (D, E) Transverse sections through the entopeduncular nucleus of the same animal as shown in (B); note the decreased cholinesterase activity at the level of the entopeduncular nucleus (E) and comb bundle (G) on the side of the lesion (×6). The thiocholine method was used in all cases. *Cd*, Caudate nucleus; *Ent*, entopeduncular nucleus; *SN*, substantia nigra; *St-N*, strionigral fibres. Reproduced with permission from Olivier *et al.* (1970).

*et al.*, 1970) together with the dopaminergic nigro-striatal fibres thus form a strio-nigro-striatal loop which could explain how impairment of neo-striatal DA metabolism can cause a "release" of cholinergic mechanisms (Larochelle *et al.*, 1971; Fig. 3.8). Furthermore, the Parkinsonian-like tremor caused by certain brain lesions can be explained in terms of

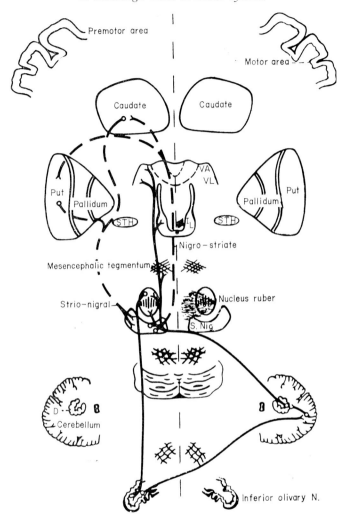

Fig. 3.8. Schematic drawing of the strio-nigro-striatal and rubro-olivo-cerebello-rubral loops. The hatched area on the right side represents the site of ventromedial tegmental lesions which produced postural tremor in monkeys. *D*, dentate nucleus; *IL*, intralaminar nuclei of the thalamus; *Put*, putamen; *S. Nig*, substantia nigra; *STH*, subthalamic nucleus; *VA* and *VL*, ventral anterior and ventrolateral nuclei of the thalamus. Reproduced with permission from Larochelle *et al.*, (1971).

involvement of the rubro-olivo-cerebello-rubral loop and the corresponding nigro-striatal mechanism (Larochelle *et al.*, 1971).

It is well known that glucose serves both as a major precursor for cerebral ACh synthesis (via formation of acetyl-CoA) and as the primary oxidative substrate of brain (see e.g. Bradford, 1968; Balazs, 1970). The following studies on tremorigenic mechanisms of the extrapyramidal system have demonstrated a relationship between cholinergic extrapyramidal function and energy metabolism. Carbon disulfide ($CS_2$) caused histological changes to occur in the globus pallidus while enhancing oxotremorine-induced tremor in the mouse (Rimski and Stern, 1967). $CS_2$ can also produce Parkinsonian-like tremor in man (Roth, 1965). This tremorigenic action of $CS_2$ could be related to an increased synthesis of cerebral ACh from acetyl-CoA-plus-choline. In support of this notion, Schuberth *et al.*, (1966) showed that brain acetyl-CoA content is increased during deep hypoxia, and $CS_2$ would be expected to cause hypoxia. Also, pertinent to the development of this idea were the findings that administration of ACh alleviated "beri-beri" (Vitamin $B_1$ deficiency; thiamine-deficiency) symptoms in pigeons (Minz and Agid, 1937), and that thiamine-deficiency causes a decrease in the degradation of pyruvate to acetyl-CoA (e.g. Fragner, 1965; McCandless and Schenker, 1968). Basing their rationale on these findings, Igić *et al.* (1968) showed that oxotremorine caused RT in normal, but not in thiamine-deficient, pigeons. Also, oxotremorine administration caused an increase in cerebral ACh content in normal, but not in "beri-beri" pigeons (Igić and Stern, 1971). This may have been due to a decrease in acetyl-CoA levels caused by thiamine deficiency (see also Heinrich *et al.*, 1973). Since the brains of "beri-beri" animals contain normal amounts of DA (Linét *et al.*, 1967) and normal or slightly-reduced amounts of ACh (Hosein *et al.*, 1966; Gubler, 1968; Cheney *et al.*, 1969; Speeg *et al.*, 1970; Stern and Igić, 1970; Igić and Stern, 1971; Heinrich *et al.*, 1973), it seems reasonable to believe that the decrease in cerebral DA which occurs in Parkinsonism (e.g. Bernheimer *et al.*, 1963) could be caused either by cellular destruction or by changes in brain ACh metabolism. Furthermore, since thiamine seems to be necessary for the tremorigenic action of oxotremorine it seems apparent that both glucose metabolism and ACh synthesis must be intact during Parkinsonism; this may perhaps be the case for all extrapyramidal dysfunctions which occur concomitantly with increased levels of cerebral ACh.

### 3.3 Convulsions

Perhaps the most dramatic of all symptoms which seem to be correlated with central cholinergic mechanisms are the severe motor seizures which are exhibited by humans suffering from some forms of epilepsy. Seizure discharges in human epileptics may arise either in discrete loci of cortical or subcortical grey matter or may be generalized phenomena at their onset. During severe motor seizures it seems likely that all areas of the neuraxis eventually become involved and that mechanisms for cerebral carbohydrate metabolism, though accelerated, remain largely intact (see Balazs, 1970). Although many studies on convulsive mechanisms have been performed, no definitive data exist to indicate a causal relationship between central cholinergic mechanisms and cryptogenic epilepsy.

A correlation between central cholinergic mechanisms and convulsions was suggested by Pope *et al.*, (1947) who found that ChE activity was increased in epileptogenic regions of human and monkey brain. In light of these data, it was suggested that the epileptogenicity of brain areas in focal epilepsy might be related to an "increased potential turnover of ACh" (see also Tower and Elliott, 1952; Guerrero-Figueroa *et al.*, 1964; Rosenburg and Echlin, 1968). Topical application of concentrated solutions of ACh ($>1\%$) to the cerebral cortex cause increases in cerebral excitability and convulsions which can be enhanced by eserine (Miller *et al.*, 1940; Chatfield and Dempsey, 1942; Arduini and Machne, 1949). Although the convulsive activity elicited by topically-applied ACh can be blocked by atropine, this effect of atropine does not occur with electrically-induced convulsions which have similar characteristics (Arduini and Machne, 1949). Therefore, the convulsions produced by ACh do not appear to be related in a primary way to central cholinergic mechanisms. Directly-applied ACh causes convulsive activity in many other regions of the brain, findings which are easily understood since iontophoretically-applied ACh excites neurones in many brain areas (see reviews by Eccles, 1964; Krnjević, 1965b; Curtis and Crawford, 1969; Phillis, 1970). In further support of this idea, it has been shown that procedures which promote increases in cerebral excitability (e.g. direct electrical stimulation) cause rapid decreases in cerebral ACh content (Richter and Crossland, 1949). Motor seizures produced by intravenously-administered pentylenetetrazol (metrazol) are also paralleled by decreases in cerebral ACh content (Crossland, 1953), and administration of convulsants to anaesthetized cats causes increases in the release of ACh from the cerebral cortex (see Chapter 6). But, these changes are more likely to be due to the induced increases in excitability and to changes in glucose metabolism than specifically to the decreased ACh content or to the drugs themselves (Stone, 1957), since seizures produced by metrazol (or strychnine) are not altered markedly by cholinergic blockade (see e.g. Herz, 1970). Other agents which produce intense motor convulsions in animals (e.g. methionine sulphoximine) do not alter cerebral ACh content or the activities of ChE or ChAc (Roa *et al.*, 1964), while cholinolytic agents used in the treatment of Parkinsonism (e.g. atropine) can cause seizures.

The hippocampus has been widely studied with regard to central seizure mechanisms since this structure has a very low threshold for

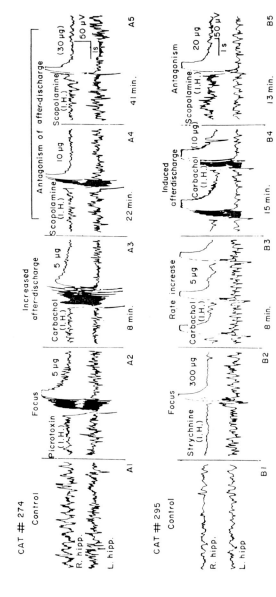

Fig. 3.9. Scopolamine antagonism of the excitatory effects of carbachol on picrotoxin- and strychnine-induced foci in cat hippocampus. Against activated picrotoxin foci, scopolamine removed the potentiation caused by carbachol (A₄), and at slightly higher doses abolished the after-discharge (A₅). The spike-wave was resistant to scopolamine. Cumulative effects of carbachol on strychnine discharge were reversed by scopolamine (B₅). Although activating the focus, carbachol potentiated the effects of scopolamine on total after-discharge component. Lapses of time after administration of each agent are indicated. Doses in parentheses are cumulative. Reproduced with permission from Baker and Benedict (1970).

seizure genesis, and since it provides, in experimental animals, a good model system for human epilepsies (especially, the psychomotor type). The hippocampus is rich in cholinergic elements (e.g. Krnjević and Silver, 1965; Lewis and Shute, 1967; Lewis *et al.*, 1967; Storm-Mathisen and Fonnum, 1969; Fonnum, 1970; Girgis, 1973; see Fig. 2.15), and its cells can be readily excited by iontophoretically-applied ACh (e.g. Brücke *et al.*, 1963; Randić and Straughan, 1965; Biscoe and Straughan, 1966) or by direct injections of ACh (e.g. MacLean and Delgado, 1953; Delgado and DeFeudis, 1969). Baker *et al.*, (1965)

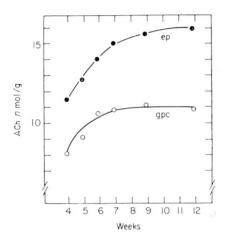

Fig. 3.10. Developmental changes in brain ACh content in a convulsive (*ep*) *v* a non-convulsive (*gpc*) strain of mouse. Note the higher ACh content of the brains of *ep* mice. Reproduced with permission from Kurokawa *et al.*, (1966).

described the production of "intermittent discharges" by intra-hippocampal injections of picrotoxin, strychnine, or *d*-tubocurarine; continuous discharge activity was also produced by intra-hippocampal carbachol or DFP (see also Baker and Benedict, 1967b, 1968a). These workers suggested that the pattern and intensity of continuous discharges in pharmacologically-established foci might involve changes in local ACh metabolism (see Baker and Benedict, 1968b). It was shown also that: (1) intra-hippocampal injections of carbachol or anti-ChE agents modified the characteristics of pharmacologically-established foci; (2) carbachol or DFP further excited these foci; (3) scopolamine reversed these effects (Baker and Benedict, 1970; see Fig. 3.9). It was concluded that a muscarinic cholinergic mechanism may be involved in the genesis of hippocampal foci. However, it should be realized that although good evidence exists to support an excitatory transmitter role

for ACh in this structure, glutamate has been shown to excite all hippocampal neurones tested (Biscoe and Straughan, 1966). Therefore,
future studies should perhaps be aimed at correlating the possible
cholinergic and amino acid mechanisms which appear to govern
hippocampal excitability and function.

Convulsive tendencies have been related to hereditary factors. Studies
performed with strains of mice which are genetically-susceptible to
convulsions have supported the view that a correlation exists between
central cholinergic mechanisms and seizures. Naruse *et al.*, (1960) found

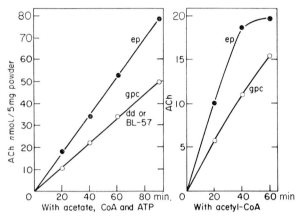

Fig. 3.11. Brain ChAc activities, estimated using either acetate, CoA plus ATP
(left) or acetyl-CoA (right) as substrate, in a convulsive (*ep*) v non-convulsive strains
of mouse. Note that the ChAc activity of the brain of the *ep* strain is about 50% higher
than that of control strains. Reproduced with permission from Kurokawa *et al.*, (1966).

that the brains of mice of the "ep" strain contain about 50% more ACh
than the brains of "control" strains, and that postural stimulation
(which causes imbalance) of "ep" mice elicits convulsions which are
correlated with decreases in their cerebral ACh content (see also
Kurokawa *et al.*, 1966; Fig. 3.10). Higher cerebral ChAc activity has also
been found in this strain although the rate of acetyl-CoA synthesis did
not differ from that of control strains (Kurokawa *et al.*, 1961; Figs 3.11
and 3.12). The "extra" ACh of the "ep" mouse brain has been characterized as an "osmotically-labile" fraction of the particle-bound compartment, and this fraction contains about twice as much ACh than is
present in "control" strains. These studies have provided evidence that a
"labile" compartment of ACh may be associated with genetically-
determined convulsive activity. It is tempting to speculate that a similar
compartment of ACh might contribute to the increased central release
of ACh which occurs during convulsions in animals which are not

genetically-susceptible to seizures (see Chapter 6). Behavioural studies performed on another strain of mice, which is genetically susceptible to convulsions by audiogenic stimuli, have indicated that cholinergic and adrenergic activities may be closely related in the genesis of audiogenic seizures and that many factors contributing to these seizures may originate in peripheral organs (Lehmann, 1970). During audiogenic seizures both the CNS and the peripheral sympathetic nervous system may relay acoustic stimuli to brain regions involved in the genesis of seizures.

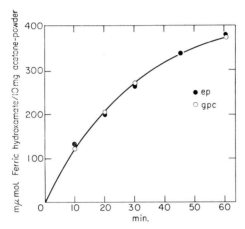

Fig. 3.12. Formation of acetyl-CoA in the brains of convulsive (*ep*) and non-convulsive (*gpc*) strains of mouse. Reproduced with permission from Kurokawa *et al.* (1966).

### 3.4 Motor Coordination: Cerebellar Function

The cerebellum is considered to be the main cerebral structure concerned with the regulation of muscular tension. This function is essential for maintaining proper control of equilibrium and posture, and for the smooth performance of voluntary movements. But, it should be remembered that the cerebellum has many other functions, and hence, it has been termed "the great modulator of neurologic function" (Snider, 1950). Relatively few studies have been conducted on the possible relationships which might exist between cerebellar mechanisms of motor coordination and its cholinergic system. However, in many studies which have been performed (e.g. those on "ep" mice (see above); those on the effects of eserine injections on "pole-jumping" behaviour (Rosecrans *et al.*, 1968)) changes in motor coordination have been produced, but the cerebellar cholinergic system has not been examined in relation to the altered function. This may be an interesting area for future research.

A number of findings support the view that cholinergic mechanisms are involved in cerebellar function. Perhaps the revulsion which must be overcome before one can become convinced that cholinergic mechanisms play significant roles in cerebellar function has stemmed from the findings that both the ACh content and ChAc activity are very low in the cerebella of various mammals (see e.g. MacIntosh, 1941; Hebb and Silver, 1956; Hebb, 1963; Phillis, 1965a, b, 1970; McCaman and Hunt, 1965; Hebb and Morris, 1969). However, cerebellar peduncles and

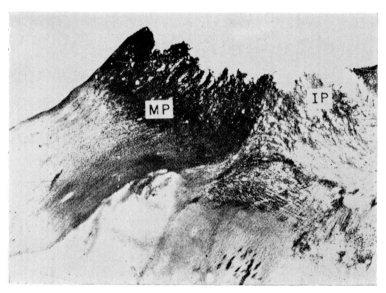

FIG. 3.13. Accumulation of AChE in the middle cerebellar peduncle (*MP*), and to a lesser extent in the inferior peduncle (*IP*) of a cat in which the peduncles were transected 4–8 days prior to death. Note the accumulation of AChE in the distended endings of the severed nerve fibres. Reproduced with permission from Phillis (1968b).

cerebellar deep nuclei do contain relatively high ChAc activities (e.g. Feldberg and Vogt, 1948; Hebb, 1961). In contrast to the findings with ACh and ChAc, the cerebellum contains high AChE activity in most areas (see e.g. Burgen and Chipman, 1951; Silver, 1967; Phillis, 1965a, 1968b; Hebb and Silver, 1970; Odutola, 1970; Figs 3.13 and 3.14). Phillis (1965a, b) found high activities of AChE in cerebellar peduncles, which when considered along with their high ChAc activities (see above) indicated that afferent fibres in the inferior and middle cerebellar peduncles and efferent fibres in the superior cerebellar peduncle may be cholinergic (Fig. 3.13). The molecular layer also contains some AChE (Austin and Phillis, 1965; Goldberg and McCaman, 1967; Odutola, 1970), and some cholinergic inter-neuronal circuits might be present in the cerebellar cortex (Phillis, 1965a). Further evidence, based on AChE staining, has indicated that some mossy fibres, parallel fibres, granule cells, association pathways and deep nuclear cells of the cat cerebellum may also be cholinergic (Phillis, 1968b; Odutola, 1970; see also Snell, 1961; Fig. 3.14). Due presumably to differences in experimental technique, Kása *et al.*, (1965) could not show that granule cells of cat cerebellum stain for AChE (see also Kása and Silver, 1969).

The lack of correlation between the amounts of ACh and ChAc activity, on the one hand, and AChE activity, on the other, does not

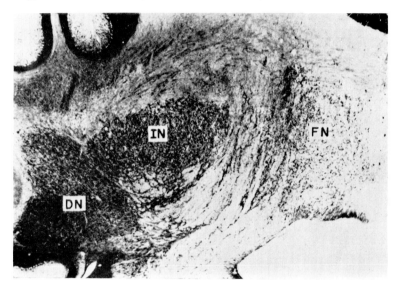

Fig. 3.14. AChE staining of cerebellar deep nuclei in the cat. *FN*, fastigial nucleus; *IN*, interpositus nucleus; *DN*, dentate nucleus. The ventrolateral area of the dentate nucleus gave a pronounced AChE reaction. Large (25–40 μ) cells are visible in all nuclei. Reproduced with permission from Phillis (1968b).

exclude the possibility that cholinergic mechanisms are involved in cerebellar function. These data could be interpreted to mean that ACh is more specific, or more potent, as a transmitter in the cerebellum than in some other brain structures so that its synthesis and degradation must be more rigorously controlled. Since ACh synthesis is linked to the main pathway for cerebral glucose metabolism, it is also possible that the cerebellum requires more acetyl-CoA for use in energy synthesis (or for the synthesis of fatty acids or steroids). This could account for the low levels of cerebellar ACh. The above findings, along with findings which have indicated that many neurones of the cerebellar cortex, and deep nuclei are excited by ACh (e.g. McCance and Phillis, 1964a, b, 1968;

Crawford *et al.*, 1966; Chapman and McCance, 1967; see reviews by Phillis, 1965b, 1970; Curtis and Crawford, 1969), that neurones of the cerebellar deep nuclei and peduncles stain for AChE (Figs 3.13 and 3.14) that ACh release from the cerebellar cortex can be increased by electrical stimulation (Mitchell, 1960; Phillis and Chong, 1965), and that cerebellar ACh is localized mainly in synaptosomal elements (e.g. Israël and Whittaker, 1965), do provide convincing evidence that cholinergic mechanisms may be involved in motor coordination and in other cerebellar functions.

### 3.5 "Circling" Behaviours

Intra-carotid injections of the potent anti-ChE agent, DFP, produced "circling" (turning) behaviours which were usually directed toward the contralateral side (e.g. Freedman and Himwich, 1949; Himwich *et al.*, 1950; Essig *et al.*, 1950; Hampson *et al.*, 1950; Himwich, 1953), but which could also be ipsilaterally directed (e.g. Essig *et al.*, 1953; Aprison *et al.*, 1954a, b). Contralateral circling has been produced in several different mammals, but was most clearly evident in monkeys. Although goats would be the most suitable animals for studying the elicitation of circling behaviour by intra-carotid administration of drugs, (see e.g. Andersson and Jewell, 1956; Reimann *et al.*, 1972) most studies have been conducted on rabbits and rats.

Aprison *et al.*, (1954a, b) showed that injections of DFP into the right common carotid arteries of rabbits caused contralateral circling most frequently, but that in some cases ipsilateral circling, or no circling, resulted. Regardless of the observed behavioural state of the animal, the AChE activities of both the caudate nucleus and the frontal cortex were decreased to a greater extent on the injected side. It was suggested that an asymmetry of AChE activity was correlated with circling behaviour and that the three different behavioural changes observed were possibly due to quantitative differences in the degree to which AChE was lowered in the right *v* left cerebral regions. These experiments, along with others in which it was shown that injections of atropine or scopolamine inhibited drug-induced circling behaviour (e.g. Himwich *et al.*, 1950; Nathan *et al.*, 1955) and that intra-carotid injections of ACh or acetyl-$\beta$-methyl-choline (Mecholyl) caused circling (Aprison *et al.*, 1956) indicated that a cholinergic system might be associated with these behavioural changes. Further experiments indicated that the caudate nuclei of contralaterally-circling rabbits contained about three times as much ACh on the right (injected) side than on the left (uninjected) side, and that the right side contained only two times as much as the left in rabbits which circled ipsilaterally (Aprison and Nathan, 1957). The ACh content of frontal cerebral cortex differed strikingly with regard to the direction of circling;

i.e. with contralateral circling the right side contained about 2·5 times as much ACh as the left side, while with ipsilateral circling the left side contained about twice as much as the right side. These workers concluded that the direction of circling which followed DFP injection was contra-lateral to the side of the cortex showing the greatest elevation in ACh, and that the rate and direction of circling were correlated with an asymmetric elevation of ACh in the cortex.

Although the above studies demonstrated, in an indirect manner, that central cholinergic mechanisms may be involved in circling behaviours, the writer feels that many criticisms apply to the techniques employed; some of these are: (1) Any retrograde flow in the right common

TABLE 7. Proportion (in per cent) of protein-bound and free radioactivity at different concentrations of $^3$H-labelled DFP in guinea pig plasma (n = 5). Reproduced with permission from Schuh (1970).

| Concentration of DFP in plasma ($M$) | Percentage of protein-bound radioactivity (Mean $\pm$ S.E.M.) | Percentage of free radioactivity (Mean $\pm$ S.E.M.) |
|---|---|---|
| $1·1 \times 10^{-7}$ | $97 \pm 2$ | $3 \pm 0·1$ |
| $2·1 \times 10^{-7}$ | $92 \pm 4$ | $8 \pm 0·35$ |
| $5·1 \times 10^{-7}$ | $67 \pm 3$ | $33 \pm 1·5$ |
| $2·1 \times 10^{-6}$ | $29 \pm 1·2$ | $71 \pm 3$ |
| $1·1 \times 10^{-5}$ | $7·4 \pm 0·4$ | $92·6 \pm 5$ |
| $10^{-4}$ | $1·5 \pm 0·08$ | $98·5 \pm 1$ |

carotid artery would allow the DFP, or other drugs administered by this route, to enter mainly the right subclavian artery for distribution in the right forelimb, or to enter the right vertebral artery for distribution into the neck region and posterior part of the brain (cerebellum, pons, other regions of the brain stem; e.g. see Sotgiu *et al.*, 1971); this could account for the variability of the observed behaviours in terms of "secondary" (peripherally-mediated) or reflex actions on the brain; (2) DFP is known to inhibit many enzymes other than AChE (e.g. dehydrogenases involved in cellular respiration; see Brooks *et al.*, 1949; Michaelis *et al.*, 1949) in most organs of the animal as well as in brain, and therefore, a complex behaviour can be at most, only vaguely correlated with the effect of this agent on the AChE-ACh system; (3) Injections made by the intra-carotid route are subject to wide animal-to-animal variation, which could also account for the variability observed; (4) The cerebro-vascular systems of mammals are subject to individual variation so that a drug should not be expected to reach the same sites of brain (or other tissues) even if injection techniques are perfectly reproducible; (5) No other substances (e.g. transmitter suspects, or other metabolites) were measured to provide control for these observations, or to test for the other effects of DFP which occurred concomitantly with its effect on the AChE-ACh system; (6) DFP, as administered, was subject to varying degrees of dilution due to individual differences in circulating blood volume and blood flow, and this agent would be expected to influence blood vessel permeability by its effects on cellular metabolism; (7) DFP is non-specifically bound to plasma proteins (Schuh, 1970; Table 7), and this could have influenced its distribution and its inhibitory action on AChE. These criticisms apply to all other studies involving this route of administration, and for this reason further research into specific brain mechanisms using these methods should be discouraged unless very strict methods of control are used.[2]

More recently, experiments have been conducted using direct injec-tions of substances into discrete areas of rat brain and with specific lesioning techniques, and more reliable circling behaviours have been produced. These studies have indicated that both ACh and dopamine (DA) are involved in circling behaviours, and that the pathways between the substantia nigra and the globus pallidus, caudate nucleus and puta-men, as well as these nuclei, are the main brain regions involved (e.g. Ungerstedt et al., 1969; Cools and Van Rossum, 1970; Arbuthnott and Crow, 1971; Costall et al., 1972). The main concept which has emerged from these studies is that the "balance" or the "level of interaction" between central cholinergic and dopaminergic mechanisms, rather than the specific stimulation or inhibition of either system, appears to be associated with the control of circling behaviours and other behaviours related to extrapyramidal function (e.g. Barbeau, 1962; Schelkunov, 1967; Klawans, 1968; Scheel-Krüger, 1970; Costall and Olley, 1971a,b; Costall et al., 1972; see §3.2, above).

Direct injections of the cholinomimetic agent, arecoline, and the major tranquilizer, haloperidol (a butyrophenone derivative which causes inhibition of dopaminergic mechanisms), into regions of the basal ganglia elicited ipsilateral circling behaviour in rats. The globus pallidus was most sensitive and substantia nigra was least sensitive to these agents,

---

[2] Most of these criticisms do not apply to the study of White (1956) in which DFP was injected directly into the right caudate nuclei of rabbits. In White's study, DFP injections always produced contralateral circling behaviour (i.e. away from the injected side) which indicates further that the variable results obtained in the studies of Aprison et al., (1954a,b) are indeed subject to these criticisms.

and the induced circling behaviour was inhibited by injections of atropine into the same sites (Costall *et al.*, 1972; see Fig. 3.3). Hence, it was suggested that either a potentiation of cholinergic mechanisms or an inhibition of dopaminergic mechanisms in these central structures caused ipsilateral circling behaviour. Support for this contention stems from earlier studies in which contralateral circling was produced by unilateral stimulation of dopaminergic mechanisms of the caudate nucleus (Ungerstedt *et al.*, 1969; Cools and Van Rossum, 1970). Also, direct injections of atropine induced contralateral circling and potentiated the ipsilateral circling caused by injections of arecoline or haloperidol

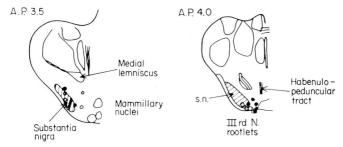

FIG. 3.15. Electrode sites (●) in the region of the substantia nigra from which electrical stimulation elicited contraversive circling behaviour in the rat. *A.P.3.5* and *A.P.4.0* are coronal sections described in the atlas of Fifkova and Marsala (1967). Reproduced with permission from Arbuthnott and Crow (1971).

into caudate-putamen or globus pallidus (Costall *et al.*, 1972). Although this analysis of circling behaviours may seem to be complete, further studies should be performed in order to reconcile these data with those which indicated that intra-caudate injections of carbachol can produce contralateral circling (Stevens *et al.*, 1961) and with the earlier studies of Himwich and coworkers (1949–58) in which ChE inhibition (by intra-carotid DFP) caused mainly contralateral circling.

Electrical stimulation of the substantia nigra or a region just rostral to it (which contains nigro-striatal fibres) can also elicit contralateral circling behaviour in rats (Arbuthnott and Crow, 1971; see Fig. 3.15); lesions placed in these same areas caused reductions in the DA content of the caudate nucleus on the lesioned side. When lesioned animals were treated with methamphetamine, they tended to turn toward the side of the lesion (Fig. 3.16). These results have supported further the notions that: (1) nigro-striatal pathways are involved in circling behaviours; (2) contralateral circling may be caused by dopaminergic stimulation (Andén, 1966; Ungerstedt *et al.*, 1969; Cools and Van Rossum, 1970); (3) inhibition of the dopaminergic system causes ipsilateral circling

(Costall *et al.*, 1972). In this connection, it is of interest that Delgado (1965) showed that contralateral circling, produced in monkeys by electrical stimulation of the red nucleus, was inhibited by chlorpromazine, an agent which is also believed to act by inhibiting central dopaminergic mechanisms. This latter finding may be correlated with the ipsilateral circling caused by systemic injections of methamphetamine into animals bearing lesions in the substantia nigra (Arbuthnott

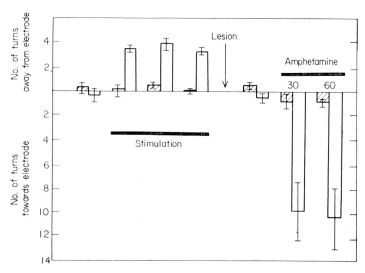

FIG. 3.16. The number of complete turns toward or away from the side of electrode placement during a 10 s period of electrical stimulation, or (after making a lesion) in 30 s periods of observation, 30 and 60 min. after administration of methamphetamine-HCl (5 mg/kg). Before the lesion, methamphetamine administration did not cause turning and after the lesion stimulation through the electrode was ineffective. *Hatched columns* represent the behaviour of rats bearing electrodes either dorsal to, or lateral to, the effective site. Reproduced with permission from Arbuthnott and Crow (1971).

and Crow, 1971; Fig. 3.16). These sympathomimetic amines have been shown to cause a release of DA.

The above findings, though subject to many technical criticisms (e.g. tissue destruction by the cannulae and electrodes; diffusion of the agents administered), do seem to provide good evidence that both cholinergic and dopaminergic mechanisms of the basal ganglia and nigro-striatal pathways are involved in circling behaviours.

*Chapter 4*

# Cholinergic Roles in Homeostatic Functions

### 4.1 Respiratory Mechanisms

Early evidence indicated that the central regulation of respiration might be mediated by cholinergic mechanisms (Dikshit, 1934a, b; Gesell *et al.*, 1943; Gesell and Hansen, 1945). Studies by Metz (1958) provided a correlation between the AChE activities of certain brain structures and the function of the central portion of a respiratory reflex arc. In further experiments on anaesthetized dogs (Metz, 1961), a significant correlation was shown to exist between a respiratory reflex response (elicited by stimulation of Hering's nerve) and the ACh contents and AChE activities of cerebral cortex, midbrain, pons, and medulla. By potentiating or inhibiting this reflex with various doses of intra-cisternally-applied tetraethyl pyrophosphate (TEPP), it was shown that cerebral ACh content was increased and that AChE activity was decreased during reflex inhibition and that opposite changes occurred during reflex potentiation (Fig. 4.1). Although ChAc activity was not correlated with the induced changes in reflex activity, it was suggested that a cholinergic mechanism might be involved in the central component of this reflex. In other studies, it was shown that HC-3, and other hemicholiniums, caused a slow, progressive failure of respiration (Long and Schueler, 1954; Schueler, 1955; Kasé and Borison, 1958; Reitzil and Long, 1959). HC-3 also interfered with the respiratory reflex response elicited by stimulation of Hering's nerve, and this action was well correlated with decreases in the ACh contents of pons and medulla (Metz, 1962; Fig. 4.2). Also, high arterial $pCO_2$ (low pH) caused small, but significant increases in ACh content of the medulla in dogs, an effect which was correlated with decreases in both medullary AChE activity and respiratory reflex response (Metz, 1964; see also Gesell and Hansen, 1945; Figs 4.3–4.5). Further studies have indicated that the release of ACh from the medulla, cerebral cortex and carotid body can be altered by subjecting animals to hypercapnia or hypoxia (Metz, 1966, 1969,

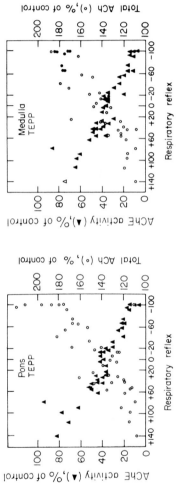

FIG. 4.1. Graphs showing relationships between acetylcholinesterase (AChE) activity (▲) and total ACh concentration (○) in the pons (*left*) and medulla (*right*) and respiratory reflex responses caused by administration of tetra-ethylpyrophosphate (TEPP) plus saline in dogs. Various doses of TEPP plus saline were administered via cisternal puncture. Data for AChE and ACh are expressed as percentage of control (taken as 100%); respiratory responses are expressed as percentage potentiation or inhibition. Each point represents one dog. From Metz (1961); reproduced with permission from the editors of *Neurology*.

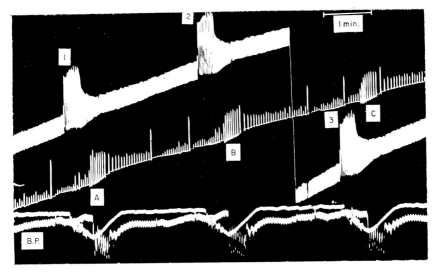

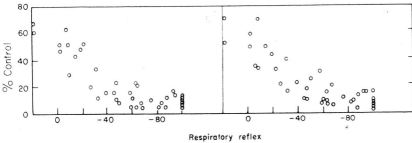

Respiratory reflex

Fig. 4.2. *Upper:* Depression of respiratory reflex responses in dogs after administration of HC-3. *1, 2* and *3* indicate steady state reflex controls elicited by electrical stimulation of Hering's nerve; *A, B* and *C* indicate responses obtained at 130, 133 and 136 min., respectively, after i.v. administration of HC-3 (0·6 mg/kg). *B.P.* = mean arterial blood pressure. Note that HC-3 induced only a slight decrease in blood pressure while causing a marked depression in respiratory reflex response. *Lower:* Relationships between total ACh concentration of the pons (*left*) and medulla (*right*), and respiratory reflex response, after administration of HC-3. Values are expressed as percentages of control level of ACh and as percentage depression of control respiratory response; each point = one dog. Reproduced with permission from the editors of the *American Journal of Physiology* (Metz, 1962).

1971a; see Chapter 6). These results have provided good support for a role of cholinergic mechanisms in central respiratory control.

## 4.2 Cardiovascular Mechanisms

Both blood pressure and heart rate may be mediated in part by cholinergic mechanisms in hypothalamic nuclei (see e.g. Brezenoff,

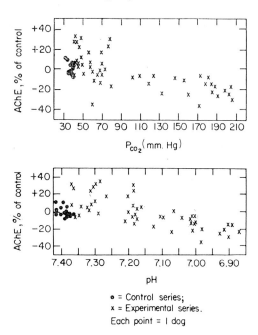

FIG. 4.3. Relationships between AChE activity of the medulla and arterial $pCO_2$ (*upper graph*) and arterial pH (*lower graph*) in anaesthetized dogs. Reproduced from Metz (1964), with permission from the editors of *Neurology*.

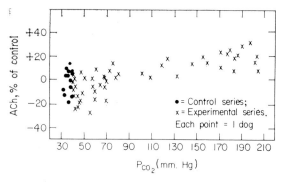

FIG. 4.4. Relationship between total ACh content of the medulla (expressed as per cent of control level) and arterial $pCO_2$ in anaesthetized dogs. Reproduced from Metz (1964), with permission from the editors of *Neurology*.

1972), by actions of ACh which were perhaps first observed in early studies by Dikshit (1934b) and Chang *et al.*, (1937a, 1938a). Hypothalamic nuclei are known to contain substantial amounts of ACh and associated enzymes (e.g. Feldberg and Vogt, 1948; Pasetto, 1952; Koelle and Geesey, 1961; Kiernon, 1964; Lederis and Livingston, 1966, 1969; see Figs 4.6 and 4.7), and changes in blood pressure have been produced by intra-ventricular injections of nicotine (Armitage and Hall, 1967;

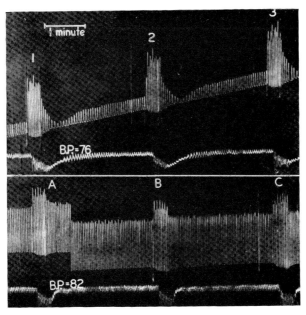

FIG. 4.5. Diminution of respiratory reflex responses by subjecting anaesthetized dogs to inhalation of high concentrations of $CO_2$; *1*, *2* and *3* are steady state reflex controls elicited by electrical stimulation of Hering's nerve; *A*, *B* and *C* are reflex responses at 24, 27 and 30 min., respectively, after administration of 22·3% $CO_2$ + 30% $O_2$; *B.P.* = mean arterial blood pressure. Reproduced from Metz (1964), with permission from the editors of *Neurology*.

Pradhan *et al.*, 1967) or carbachol (Brezenoff and Jenden, 1969, 1970). Since the hypotensive responses evoked by intra-hypothalamic injections of muscarinic agents (e.g. oxotremorine) were blocked by prior central injections of atropine, this effect may involve muscarinic receptors (Brezenoff and Wirecki, 1970). Intra-hypothalamic injections of *d*-tubocurarine have been shown to evoke pressor responses in cats (Fletcher and Pradhan, 1969), and in the recent studies of Brezenoff (1972) direct injections of carbachol or neostigmine into the posterior or ventromedial nuclei of rat hypothalamus consistently produced increases in both systemic blood pressure and heart rate (Table 8). In Brezenoff's work, cardiovascular responses evoked by injections of eserine or edrophonium into the posterior hypothalamus were similar, but more variable, than those produced by carbachol or neostigmine; injections of carbachol into dorsomedial or pre-mammillary areas of the

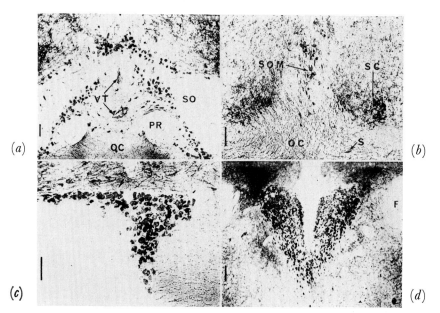

Fig. 4.6. Transverse sections of guinea pig hypothalamus stained for AChE: *a*, note strong AChE activity in tuft of blood vessels (*VI*) close to rostral limit of supraoptic nucleus; *b*, lateral supraoptic nucleus; *c*, midline component of supraoptic nucleus and supra-chiasmatic neuropil; note S, cell of supraoptic nucleus in optic chiasma; *d*, paraventricular nucleus at fairly rostral level. PR, preoptic recess; SO, supraoptic nucleus; OC, optic chiasma; SOM, midline component of the supraoptic nucleus; SC, supra-chiasmatic neuropil; F, columns of the fornix; P, paraventricular nucleus. Scale bars: a–c, 100 $\mu$; d, 200 $\mu$. Reproduced with permission from Cottle and Silver (1970).

hypothalamus caused bradycardia and hypotensive responses (Table 8). These pharmacological studies support the hypothesis that central cardiovascular control may be mediated, at least in part, by cholinergic mechanisms.

### 4.3 Anti-Diuretic Hormone (Vasopressin) and Oxytocin Secretion

By definition, "neurosecretory cells" of the supraoptic (SO) and paraventricular (PV) nuclei of the hypothalamus may serve a dual role:

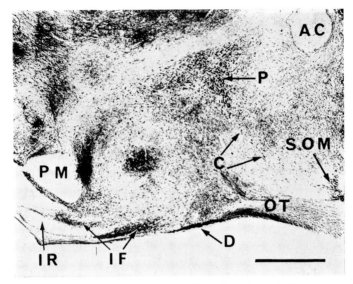

Fig. 4.7. AChE activity in a parasaggital section through the paraventricular nucleus, supraoptic midline and infundibular nuclei of guinea pig hypothalamus. AC, anterior commissure; C, cells forming continuity between paraventricular and supraoptic nuclei; D, diffusus component of supraoptic nucleus; IF, infundibular nucleus; IR, infundibular recess; OT, optic tract; P, paraventricular nucleus; PM, pre-mammillary recess; SOM, midline component of supraoptic nucleus; Scale bars: 1 mm. Thiocholine technique. Reproduced with permission from Cottle and Silver (1970).

TABLE 8. Cardiovascular responses (Mean $\pm$ S.E.) to injections of carbachol or neostigmine into the posterior hypothalamic (PH), ventromedial (VM), dorsomedial (DM) or pre-mammillary (PM) nuclei. Reproduced with permission from Brezenoff (1972).

| Drug (3 $\mu$g) | Injection site (n) | BP (mm Hg)[a] Control | Drug | Heart rate (beats/min.) Control | Drug |
|---|---|---|---|---|---|
| Carbachol | PH, VM (15) | $\dfrac{145.0 \pm 5.0}{103.0 \pm 6.2}$ | $\dfrac{183.5 \pm 3.9^{b}}{142.5 \pm 4.0^{b}}$ | $380.0 \pm 13.4$ | $418.5^{d}$ |
| Carbachol | DM, PM (8) | $\dfrac{153.3 \pm 4.4}{105.8 \pm 5.8}$ | $\dfrac{128.3 \pm 8.0^{c}}{78.3 \pm 9.2^{b}}$ | $369.2 \pm 14.2$ | $281.7 \pm 15.1^{c}$ |
| Neostigmine | All sites (11) | $\dfrac{135.5 \pm 5.3}{89.5 \pm 4.9}$ | $\dfrac{183.2 \pm 7.1^{b}}{137.2 \pm 4.9^{b}}$ | $371.4 \pm 16.5$ | $418.6 \pm 11.7^{c}$ |

[a] Systolic/diastolic.
[b] $p < 0.001$.
[c] $p < 0.01$.
[d] Not significant ($0.05 < p < 0.1$). Numbers of experiments (n) are in parentheses.

(1) transmission of nervous impulses, and; (2) elaboration of the endo-crine secretions, anti-diuretic hormone (ADH) and oxytocin. As stated in the preceding section, substantial amounts of ACh and related enzymatic activities have been found in mammalian hypothalami. Also, both ChAc (Feldberg and Vogt, 1948; Feldberg, 1949) and AChE (Abrahams *et al.*, 1957; Cottle and Silver, 1970) activities have been demonstrated in the SO and PV nuclei (see Figs 4.6 and 4.7).

After Dikshit (1934a, b, c, 1935) showed that injections of ACh into the hypothalamus or cerebral ventricles of cats produced central effects, it was shown that stimulation of the central end of the severed vagus nerve of the dog evoked a release of "pitressin" (ADH) and an oxytocic principle from the posterior pituitary and that these effects were corre-lated with a release of ACh into the cerebral circulation as well as with a delayed "pressor" response (Chang *et al.*, 1937a, b, c, 1938a, b). (Since at least in man, several hundred times as much ADH is required to obtain a "pressor" (vasoconstrictor) action than to produce maximal diuresis (Brazeau, 1971), only its diuretic action will be discussed here.) Pickford (1939) then showed, using un-anaesthetized, atropinized dogs, that intravenously-injected ACh caused a temporary inhibition of water-induced diuresis; in thirsty dogs, ACh injections caused a diuresis. From these actions of ACh, along with the finding that these effects of ACh could be abolished by removing the posterior pituitary, Pickford concluded that ACh promoted a release of ADH from the posterior pituitary to the blood-stream by a central action. Intra-carotid injections of ACh also inhibited water-induced diuresis by an action that was enhanced by eserine (Pickford and Watt, 1951). Directly-injected ACh, DFP, or eserine into the SO nuclei of anaesthetized dogs also caused this effect (Pickford, 1947; Duke *et al.*, 1950). Duke and Pickford (1951) showed further that administration of adrenaline, together with or just prior to intravenous injection of ACh, prevented the inhibitory action of ACh on water-induced diuresis in about half of the animals studied; more rarely, adrenaline potentiated the action of ACh, or had no effect. These were the first studies which indicated that both cholinergic and adrenergic mechanisms might regulate the central release of ADH (see review by Bisset, 1968). Although variability was encountered in these studies, due to the systemic route of injection and to individual differences in the experimental animals, a good element of control was provided by the demonstration that injections of ACh directly into the mammillary bodies or lateral hypothalamus did not inhibit water-induced diuresis (Pickford, 1947). In anaesthetized female dogs, treated with stiboestrol, direct injections of eserine or DFP into the SO nuclei caused prolonged increases of spontaneous uterine activity (Abrahams and Pickford, 1956). Milk-ejection responses, similar to those produced by oxytocin, were also produced in lactating bitches by intravenous or intra-carotid injections of ACh (Pickford, 1960; Brooks *et al.*, 1966). Hence, it seems likely that cholinergic mechanisms are associated with the secretion of both ADH and oxytocin from the posterior pituitary.

It is particularly noteworthy that in many of the studies mentioned above, (e.g. those of Pickford, 1939) the animals had been atropinized in order to prevent peripheral (muscarinic) actions of the injected ACh. This indicated that the observed effects of ACh on the SO and PV nuclei were nicotinic, since atropine would be expected to enter the brain under these conditions. The nicotinic nature of these responses was supported further by studies in which it was shown that nicotine caused an anti-diuretic action in rats by an effect which could be blocked by hypophysectomy (Burn *et al.*, 1945). Also, intravenously-administered nicotine or inhalation of cigarette smoke is known to produce anti-diuresis in man (e.g. Walker, 1949; Burn and Grewal, 1951; Chalmers and Lewis, 1951; Bisset and Lee, 1958). Nicotine also caused a release of both ADH and oxytocin into the circulation in rats (Walker, 1957; Bisset and Walker, 1957; Grewal *et al.*, 1962).

Several electrophysiological investigations on single unit activity in the SO and PV nuclei have supported the contention that ACh may be a transmitter mediating the afferent input to neurosecretory cells. However, it should be remembered that the secretory activity of these cells may be modulated by the combined actions of ACh and catecholamines (see Bisset, 1968; Barker *et al.*, 1971a, b). Cross and Green (1959) showed, in lightly-anaesthetized rabbits, that the firing rates of SO neurones were usually accelerated by intra-carotid injections of hyper-osmotic solutions of NaCl or glucose, but that PV neurones were inhibited; many neurones of neighbouring hypothalamic nuclei also responded to hyper-osmotic stimuli. It is noteworthy that the majority of neurones responding to hyper-osmotic stimuli in the studies of Cross and Green (1959) did not respond to tactile, visual, or auditory stimuli. Dyball and Koizumi (1969) showed that the excitation of SO and PV cells of rats, caused by stimulation of the central end of the severed vagus nerve, or by intra-carotid injections of $CaCl_2$, was correlated with a release of both ADH and oxytocin (see also Lederis, 1962). Dyball (1971) showed further that intra-carotid injections of hyper-osmotic solutions of NaCl excited some antidromically-identified, neurosecretory cells of the SO nucleus, but inhibited others. Although less PV than SO cells were excited by hyper-osmotic stimuli in Dyball's study, the concentration of oxytocin in blood increased about 8-fold while that of ADH increased only about 2·7-fold; hormonal secretion outlasted the induced increases in firing rate of these cells.

Many problems remain unsolved with regard to the proposed

cholinergic mechanism of neurosecretion from the posterior pituitary. In order to explain fully these secretory phenomena, the following points should perhaps be considered: (1) SO neurones may interconnect with PV neurones. Evidence that this may occur has been derived from anatomical (Bargmann, 1949; Cottle and Silver, 1970; see Fig. 4.7) and electrophysiological (Yamashita *et al.*, 1970) studies, and therefore, it seems possible that neither ADH nor oxytocin are released selectively in the intact animal; (2) "Osmoreceptor" neurones (Verney, 1947) may

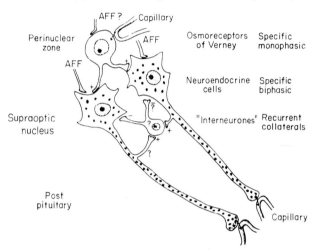

FIG. 4.8. Vincent and Hayward's schematic interpretation of possible cellular connections in the osmoreceptor-supraoptic nuclear complex of the monkey. The "osmoreceptors" of Verney are distinct neurones which respond "specifically" to an osmotic stimulus with a "monophasic" discharge which is transferred directly to neuroendocrine cells of the supraoptic nucleus (NSO). It was suggested further that supraoptic neuroendocrine cells respond to an osmotic stimulus with an initial acceleration discharge, due to the synaptic driving by the "osmoreceptors", followed quickly by an inhibitory phase possibly due to recurrent collateral activation of "interneurones" or via direct action on these neuroendocrine cells with a slow postsynaptic potential. These supraoptic cells show a specific "biphasic" discharge to an osmotic stimulus. AFF, afferent fibre connections; +, excitatory synaptic action; —, inhibitory synaptic action; ?, and unknown entity. Reproduced with permission from Vincent and Hayward (1970).

relay osmotic signals either to "specific" or to "non-specific osmosensitive" cells during the secretory responses, as has been shown recently in monkeys (Hayward and Vincent, 1970); (3) The anatomical explanation for the effects observed in the above-mentioned studies may involve pathways of "recurrent inhibition" with regard to the responses of SO neurosecretory cells (Hayward and Vincent, 1970; Vincent and Hayward, 1970; Dreifuss and Kelly, 1972a; Fig. 4.8).

In iontophoretic studies performed on anaesthetized cats, it has been shown that SO neurosecretory cells can be depressed by nor-adrenaline (NA), and that ACh can elicit both muscarinic depressant and nicotinic exitatory actions (Barker *et al.*, 1971a, b; see Fig. 4.9). About 90 % of the "responsive" cells were depressed by NA, about 84 % were depressed by ACh, and about 16 % were excited by ACh, and all responses to NA and ACh could be shown in the same neurosecretory cell (Barker *et al.*, 1971a, b). In these studies, serotonin (5-HT) and dopamine (DA) also depressed

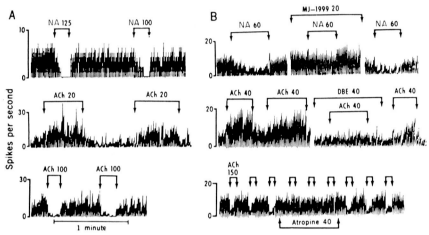

FIG. 4.9. Responses of supraoptic neurones to ACh and nor-adrenaline (NA). A, NA-induced depression and ACh-induced excitation and depression of activity in three different antidromically-identified neurosecretory cells. B, *top:* blockade of NA-induced depression by the β-adrenergic blocking agent, MJ-1999; *middle:* antagonism of ACh-induced excitation by dihydro-β-erythroidine (DBE); *bottom:* blockade of ACh-induced depression by atropine. Numbers next to drug abbreviations indicate iontophoretic currents (*n*-Amp). Reproduced with permission from Barker *et al.* (1971b).

the activity of responsive cells, and NA depressed excitatory responses caused by ACh. Studies on SO neurosecretory cells of rats (Dreifuss and Kelly, 1972b) supported the finding that the excitatory action of ACh on these cells is mainly nicotinic since very large doses of atropine were required to block this action and since it was more readily blocked by the nicotinic antagonist, dihydro-β-erythroidine. Dreifuss and Kelly showed no obvious depressant actions of ACh on the cells tested. The disparity between the results obtained by these two groups of workers regarding the depressant effect of ACh may have been due to species differences and/or to the use of different anaesthetics. Iontophoretic application of ACh excited 91 % of the antidromically-identified neurosecretory cells of the PV nucleus of rabbit hypothalamus, while NA inhibited 83% of these cells (Moss *et al.*, 1972). In this study, it was shown that opposite effects were produced on PV cells which were not antidromically invaded; i.e. 76% were depressed by ACh and 81% were excited by NA. It was suggested that the effects of ACh might be mediated by both nicotinic and muscarinic receptors, and perhaps by a "mixed type" receptor.

Perhaps the major conclusion to be derived from this research on transmitter modulation of neurosecretion from the posterior pituitary is that the secretion of both ADH and oxytocin are correlated with ACh-sensitive neuronal activity in neurosecretory cells in SO and PV nuclei. But, there exists considerable overlap both in the effects or peripherally-applied stimuli which stimulate these secretory processes and in the possible transmitter mechanisms involved in producing the secretions. It seems apparent that both cholinergic and adrenergic mechanisms may play significant roles, but other possible transmitter systems, such as those utilizing GABA and glutamate, may also be associated with these phenomena (see Moss *et al.*, 1972).

### 4.4 Temperature Regulation

Cholinergic mechanisms may also be involved in the central regulation of body temperature. A thermoregulatory role for the hypothalamus was indicated in the early history of its study (see e.g. review by Cooper, 1966). Results of more recent studies have indicated that ACh, serotonin (5-HT), nor-adrenaline (NA) and adrenaline (ADR) may all be involved in the regulation of body temperature. However, the data supporting the hypothesis that all of these transmitter suspects might be implicated in the central control of temperature have usually been obtained by injecting very large amounts of these substances directly into the brain or CSF, and are also subject to marked species variation. After the suggestion by Brodie and Shore (1957) that catecholamines of the hypothalamus might be involved in temperature regulation, Feldberg and Myers (1964, 1965), using intra-ventricular or intra-hypothalamic injections, found that 5-HT caused increases, and that NA and ADR caused decreases, in the body temperatures of unanaesthetized cats. Experiments with rabbits (Cooper *et al.*, 1965) and sheep (Bligh, 1966) yielded exactly opposite results. When injections were made directly into the anterior hypothalamus (see e.g. Feldberg and Myers, 1965), the amounts of test substances (e.g. NA) injected were usually greater than the amount of amine endogenous to the whole hypothalamus.

Perhaps the first indication that a cholinergic mechanism might be involved in central thermoregulatory responses derives from the studies of Henderson and Wilson (1936) in which it was shown that "shivering" could be elicited in man by intra-ventricular injections of ACh. Later,

Feldberg and Malcolm (1959) showed that intra-ventricular injections of *d*-tubocurarine (*d*-TC) caused "tremor-like" responses in anaesthetized cats, which resembled shivering. By perfusing selective portions of the cerebral ventricular system, it was shown further that shivering elicited by *d*-TC was likely to be due to its action on the hypothalamus (Carmichael *et al.*, 1962). Although Cooper *et al.*, (1965) could not produce any effect on body temperature by injecting ACh or ACh-plus-eserine mixtures directly into the anterior hypothalamus of rabbits, Myers and Yaksh (1969) reported that large amounts of ACh-plus-eserine (2–25 $\mu$g) or carbachol (0·4–2 $\mu$g) injected into various areas of the hypothalamus of monkeys usually produced hyperthermia. In other studies, intra-ventricular injections of ACh or ACh-plus-eserine (5–50 $\mu$g) into rats usually caused hyperthermia, which was measured as a long-lasting increase in colonic temperature (Myers and Yaksh, 1968).

In support of the results of Myers and Yaksh (1968), Avery (1970, 1971) showed that a dose-dependent increase in colonic temperature followed pre-optic injections of 3–8 $\mu$g carbachol. But, on the other hand, injections of large (20–50 $\mu$g) amounts of ACh into the pre-optic/anterior hypothalamic area of rats have also been shown to cause an "immediate" fall in both hypothalamic and body temperature (Beckman and Carlisle, 1969; Kirkpatrick and Lomax, 1970). In an effort to resolve these conflicting sets of data, Crawshaw (1973) monitored thermoregulatory responses to bilateral injections of 50 $\mu$g ACh into the pre-optic/anterior hypothalamic area of rats. His results indicated that ACh elicited immediate "heat-loss" responses. Since the maximum decrease in hypothalamic temperature occurred within a few minutes after injection of ACh, this response could not have been observed by Myers and Yaksh (1968) who monitored colonic temperature at 15 and 30 min. post-injection. At these later times, Crawshaw (1973) found that there occurred a slow increase in temperature. It should also be noted that the "heat-loss" response to ACh was obscured if rats were active (aroused) during the post-injection period. Arousal level could have been increased by the procedures of Myers and Yaksh (1968) which included the insertion of thermometers into the anal orifices of rats.

Since the mammalian hypothalamus contains only about 2 $\mu$g ACh/g, fresh weight (see e.g. refs. in Phillis, 1970), the above studies have not provided good evidence for a role of ACh in thermoregulation. However, in un-anaesthetized mice, subcutaneous injections of the cholinomimetic agent, arecoline, caused hypothermia (Nikki, 1969) and prevented halothane-induced shivering (Nikki, 1968). These effects of arecoline could have been centrally-mediated and muscarinic since they were inhibited by systemic injections of atropine, but not by N-methyl-atropine. Systemic, or intra-cerebral injections of other cholinergic drugs (e.g. eserine, oxotremorine) have also been shown to lower body temperature in rats (Maickel *et al.*, 1964; Lomax and Jenden, 1966; Zetler, 1968).

The results presented above lend some indirect support to the contention that a central cholinergic system may be involved in temperature regulation, but the relationships which may exist between this system and other possible transmitter systems in the hypothalamus remain rather completely obscure. A major pitfall was encountered when attempting to interpret the data on the effects of intra-hypothalamic injections of ACh and other substances (e.g. those of Myers and Yaksh, 1968, 1969) since the effects obtained with such large amounts of injected substance were perhaps not at all "physiological". Also, evoked changes in body temperature have been shown to be variable and not always predictable, with respect to sites of injection of cholinergic drugs, in diencephalic and mesencephalic regions of cat's brain (see Rudy and Wolf, 1972). A review of neural processes involved in thermoregulation has recently appeared (Hensel, 1973).

*Chapter 5*

# Cholinergic Roles in Motivated Behaviours, Emotion, Learning and Memory

## 5.1 Ingestive Behaviours

### *A. Introduction*

It is generally maintained that structures of the diencephalon and limbic system are associated with the regulation of food and water intake. The hypothalamus seems to be most significantly associated with these behaviours. Results obtained by direct application of cholinergic or anti-cholinergic agents to discrete brain structures have led to the hypothesis that the lateral hypothalamus (LH) and several other limbic structures are involved in a "cholinergically-mediated thirst circuit" which can activate drinking behaviour in rats (e.g. Grossman, 1960, 1962a, b; Fisher and Coury, 1962, 1964). Interestingly, this "thirst circuit" corresponds anatomically to the system of limbic structures which has been associated with emotionality and motivated behaviours (Papez, 1937; MacLean, 1958; Nauta, 1963; Fig. 5.1). Since the anatomical representation of drinking behaviour is in considerable overlap with that for other behaviours, simple anatomical (or functional) substrates for these behaviours perhaps do not exist. Hence, ingestive behaviours may be considered to be motivated behaviours. Many studies have been conducted in an effort to define the anatomical circuitry of the central "drinking" and "feeding" systems, and to define the transmitter processes which may underlie their activation and inhibition.

Early findings made with techniques of brain lesioning and electrical stimulation, led to the belief that LH areas were associated with "feeding" ("eating") behaviour and that the ventromedial hypothalamic area (VMH) was a "satiety centre" (e.g. Anand and Brobeck, 1951;

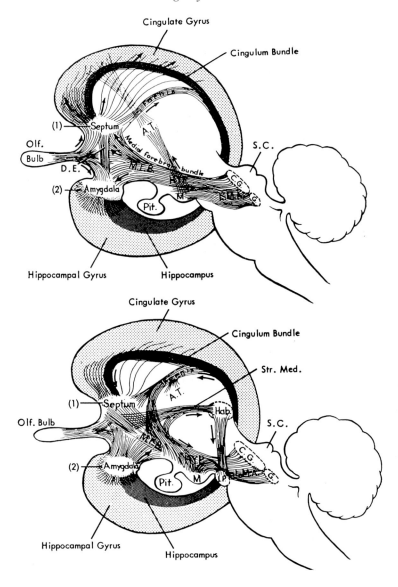

FIG. 5.1. MacLean's schemata for the organization of the limbic system. *Upper:*
Projections by a variety of divergent pathways from olfactory bulb and brain stem
into the limbic system. *Lower:* Limbic outflow by way of the fornix, medial forebrain
bundle and habenulo-peduncular tract to the brain stem. The anteriomedial region
of this circuit, in the vicinity of the septum (1), has been identified by MacLean as
relating predominantly to "survival of the species". The anteriolateral region, in the
vicinity of the amygdala (2), has been identified as relating predominately to "survival
of the individual". Reproduced with permission from MacLean (1958).

Delgado and Anand, 1953; Smith, 1956; Miller, 1960). Later it was suggested that this dual "feeding system" might be modulated significantly by interconnected limbic structures (e.g. Stevenson, 1964), in a fashion similar to that of the "drinking system". Thus, it became apparent that the "feeding" and "drinking" systems were perhaps in considerable anatomical overlap with one another and that the main anatomical areas concerned (e.g. LH, VMH) were also associated with emotional (affective) reactions (see e.g. Wheatley, 1944; Hess, 1949) as well as with hormonal functions. It seems unlikely that two distinct networks exist for the modulation of feeding and drinking behaviours, as has been recently proposed (e.g. Coury, 1967). However, it does seem possible that the anatomical substrates for ingestive behaviours are related intimately to those subserving affective and motivational behaviours, as has been suggested recently for VMH function in rats (Grossman, 1966a).

It was originally proposed, from data obtained with intra-cerebral injections of cholinergic agonists (e.g. carbachol) and antagonists (e.g. atropine) in rats, that ACh might be involved in the central mediation of drinking behaviour, and that an adrenergic limbic circuit might be associated with food intake (Grossman, 1960; see also, Grossman, 1962a, b; Fisher and Coury, 1962, 1964; Stein and Seifter, 1962; Miller *et al.*, 1964; Levitt and Fisher, 1966). However, when experiments were conducted with higher mammals, the results began to differ. For example food and water intake in Rhesus monkeys could not be explained simply in terms of cholinergic and adrenergic mechanisms (e.g. Myers, 1969). In all cases, other parameters (e.g. dose of drug; exact implantation site; type of injection—solid or solution; hormonal factors), as well as species differences, entered into the interpretations of the observed effects (see §5.1, D, below). Another aspect worthy of consideration is the types of stimuli which have been used to evoke these behaviours. For example, what portion of the feeding and drinking responses might be due to mechanisms related to defence, prey-killing, or to emotional expression? What are the physiological stimuli and are these distinct? Surely these stimuli will depend to a great extent on the species of animal examined, their ages, and their environments both before and during experiments. These factors make it extremely difficult to draw conclusions from results obtained in different laboratories. Also, the physiological stimuli associated with ingestive behaviours are complex and certainly not well understood at present, and feedback mechanisms in diencephalic structures may play important roles (Morgane, 1964). The intense anatomical overlap between hypothalamic areas associated with "rage", "attack", and sexual behaviours and those associated with ingestive behaviours indicates that these behaviours may all be interrelated. However, the diffuse natures of these systems as well as their extensive anatomical overlap make this an interesting and very challenging area for further study.

### B. Drinking Behaviour

By far, most studies on drinking behaviour have been conducted on rats. Cholinergic stimulation with carbachol (carbamycholine) of many sites within the hypothalamus, thalamus, pre-optic region, medial septum, cingulate gyrus and hippocampus has elicited drinking behaviour in satiated rats (e.g. Grossman, 1960, 1962a, b; 1964; Fisher and Coury,

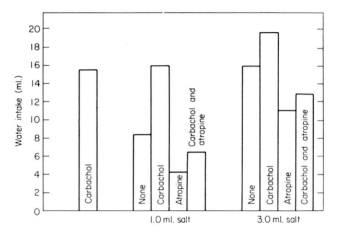

Fig. 5.2. Interaction of chemical brain stimulation (of lateral septal nucleus or anterior thalamic region) and salt-induced drinking behaviour in the rat. The bar on the left indicates the mean water intake following implantation of crystalline carbachol (2–3 μg) into positive "drinking" sites. The next two groups of bars show mean water intakes following 1·0- or 3·0-ml subcutaneous injections of hypertonic salt solution (15% NaCl + 2·5% procaine-HCl; procaine was used to reduce irritation from the salt); alone (None or in combination with each of the three intra-cerebral implantations. Note that intra-cerebrally-administered atropine exerted a much more pronounced effect on carbachol-elicited drinking than on salt induced drinking. Atropine was administered bilaterally, and atropine and carbachol were administered into contralateral sites. Reproduced with permission from Levitt and Buerger (1970).

1962; Miller *et al.*, 1964; Miller, 1965; Quartermain and Miller, 1966; Levitt *et al.*, 1970; Krikstone and Levitt, 1970). Carbachol-induced drinking has been inhibited by peripheral (e.g. Grossman, 1962a) or central (e.g. Grossman, 1962b; Levitt and Fisher, 1966) injection of atropine, but atropine produced a much greater inhibitory effect on carbachol-induced drinking than on salt- or deprivation-induced water intake (e.g. Krikstone and Levitt, 1970; Levitt and Buerger, 1970; Fig.

5.2). Drinking responses have been elicited by implantation of crystalline carbachol (e.g. Grossman, 1960, 1964) or by injection of carbachol in solution (e.g. Miller *et al.*, 1964; Levitt, 1970).

Studies by Levitt and Boley (1970) indicated that a high correlation exists among sites in the limbic system from which carbachol and eserine elicited drinking and that eserine-induced drinking was antagonized by atropine in all sites tested (see Fig. 5.3). In other studies with anti-ChE agents, Winson and Miller (1970) showed that injections of eserine

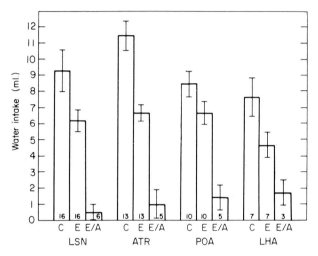

Fig. 5.3. Drinking elicited by injection of eserine or carbachol into various regions of rat brain, and the inhibition of eserine-induced drinking by atropine. LSN, lateral septal nucleus; ATR, anterior thalamic region; POA, preoptic area; LHA, lateral hypothalamic area; C = carbachol; E = eserine; E/A = eserine injection into the site indicated and atropine injection into another "drinking" site. Vertical lines at tops of bars indicate S.E.M.; numbers of observations are given in the bottom of each bar. Reproduced with permission from Levitt and Boley (1970).

directly into the pre-optic area caused water-satiated rats to drink within 60 min. after injection, but not beyond that time, while injections of DFP caused drinking for times up to 210 min. (see also Miller and Chien, 1968). These workers suggested that the relatively rapid reversibility of eserine's action was due to a decrease in its concentration at the injection site, while the slower cessation of DFP action might have been due to re-synthesis of an isoenzyme of AChE, or to spontaneous reactivation of AChE.

Miller *et al.*, (1964) showed that certain quantities of carbachol ($2 \cdot 7 \times 10^{-10} - 24 \times 10^{-10}$ mol) caused reliable drinking behaviour when injected into rat hypothalamic areas, while higher doses elicited less drinking, lethargy, and then convulsions (see Fig. 5.4). Carbachol

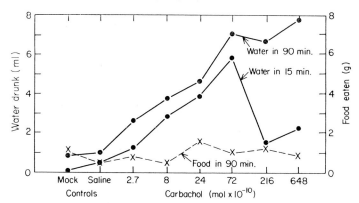

Fig. 5.4. Effects of direct injections of different amounts of carbachol into the region of the ventromedial hypothalamic nucleus on feeding and drinking behaviour in the satiated rat. Reproduced with permission from Miller *et al.* (1964).

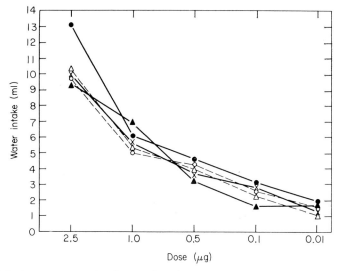

Fig. 5.5. Average water intake as a function of site of cerebral stimulation for five different amounts of carbachol: ●—●, septum; ○—○, hypothalamus; ▲—▲, thalamus; △—△, hippocampus-fornix; ×—×, corpus callosum. Reproduced with permission from Levitt *et al.* (1970).

did not produce appreciable feeding behaviour at any of the amounts used in these studies. These results indicated that certain hypothalamic areas might be related more specifically to drinking behaviour than to convulsions. Also, it has been shown that central application of atropine to one cholinergically-activated drinking site inhibited carbachol- or eserine-induced drinking at a second such site (Levitt and Fisher, 1966;

Levitt and Boley, 1970). However, these effects of atropine could have been caused by its diffusion to the second site. Levitt *et al.*, (1970) showed that injections of carbachol into rat limbic areas induced drinking behaviour after about 3·5 min., but that with crystalline implantations drinking took about 6·5 min. to occur. Interestingly, the dipsogenic effect of carbachol was not localized at any particular limbic area studied (see

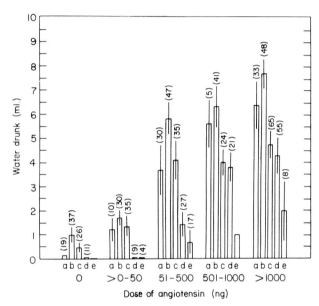

Fig. 5.6. Relationship between mean amounts of water drunk and intra-cranial dose of angiotensin in the rat. Results for all animals have been grouped together according to the range of doses used and the anatomical locus of the cannula tip. Note the decrease in sensitivity as the site of injection is moved from septal region (a), preoptic region (b) and anterior hypothalamic area (c) to lateral hypothalamic area (d) and ventromedial hypothalamic area (e). Vertical lines on bars represent ±1 S.E.M.; numbers of observations in parentheses. Reproduced with permission from Epstein *et al.*, (1970).

Fig. 5.5). In rats, Myers and Yaksh (1968) found that intra-ventricular injections of ACh or eserine did not induce drinking behaviour. Lovett and Singer (1971), on the other hand, showed that intra-ventricular injections of carbachol elicited drinking in both satiated and deprived rats.

Angiotensin, renin, and aldosterone all seem to be involved in "normal" drinking behaviour (e.g. Fitzsimons, 1966; Wolf and Handal, 1966; Fitzsimons and Simons, 1968, 1969). Crystalline angiotensin (like carbachol) increased fluid intake when implanted in the rat anterior hypothalamus, but this did not occur in the VMH (Hendler and Blake, 1969). Epstein *et al.*, (1970) showed further that the structures of rat brain which were most sensitive to the dipsogenic action of angiotensin were anterior hypothalamus, pre-optic region and septum (see Fig. 5.6). Angiotensin was also shown to be a more potent dipsogen than carbachol (e.g. Grossman, 1960), hypertonic saline (e.g. Andersson, 1953) or nor-adrenaline (e.g. Booth, 1968). It is noteworthy that carbachol seems to produce drinking reliably only in rats, whereas angiotensin affects a number of species (see refs in Epstein *et al.*, 1970). Release of angiotensin from the kidney might be a major factor associated with the central regulation of naturally-occurring drinking behaviour; i.e. the drinking which is induced by thirst or by extra- or intra-cellular dehydration (e.g. Fitzsimons, 1961, 1966, 1969; Stricker, 1966). A comprehensive review of studies concerning the central effects of angiotensin in relation to mechanisms of hydration has appeared (see Severs and Daniels-Severs, 1973).

Drinking behaviour has also been elicited by subcutaneous injections of hypertonic salt solutions (Wayner and Reamanis, 1958) by a mechanism which can be inhibited by peripherally-injected atropine (De-Weid, 1966). However, injections of carbachol into brain structures increased fluid intake to levels above that caused by salt alone (Levitt and Buerger, 1970; Fig. 5.2), which could mean that the mechanism for naturally-induced drinking is not exclusively cholinergic (or that carbachol-induced drinking does not mimic "natural" drinking). Also, Miller (1965) reported that intra-cerebral administration of ACh, or carbachol, in addition to causing satiated rats to drink, facilitated their performance of thirst-motivated, learned behaviours, stimulated their renal re-absorption of water (Fig. 5.7) and caused marked increases in their blood glucose levels (Fig. 5.8). Therefore, anti-diuretic hormone (ADH) may be involved in carbachol-induced drinking in rats. By spaced presentation of food, a phenomenon termed "schedule-induced polydipsia" has been produced in rats (Falk, 1961), Burks and Fisher (1970) tested the sensitivity of this behaviour to atropine. Intra-peritoneal injections of atropine inhibited schedule-induced polydipsia in a dose-dependent fashion, which indicated that this phenomenon may be mediated, at least in part, by central cholinergic pathways. In other studies, it was shown that bilateral septal lesions increased water intake by rats (Harvey and Hunt, 1965; Blass and Hanson, 1970), and this effect appeared to be correlated with a significant decrease in cerebral ACh content (Sorensen and Harvey, 1971). However, in recent studies by Pepeu *et al.*, (1973) it was shown that though septal lesions caused a pronounced reduction of brain ACh, no change occurred in daily water consumption (see also Grace, 1968; Besch and Van Dyne, 1969; Pepeu *et al.*, 1971).

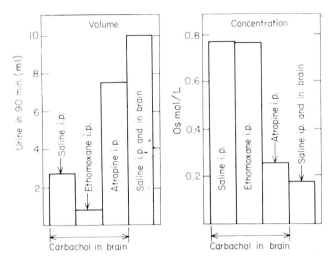

FIG. 5.7. Effects of injections of carbachol into the lateral hypothalamus of the un-anaesthetized rat. As shown, carbachol caused a reduction in the volume and in increase in the concentration of the urine by an action which was antagonized by intra-peritoneal injections of atropine, but not by the adrenergic blocking agent, ethomoxane, or by the saline vehicle. Data of Miller and Chien; reproduced with permission from Miller (1965).

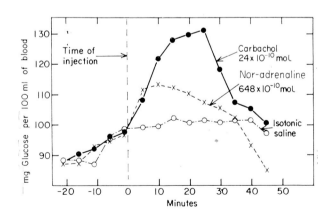

FIG. 5.8. Effects on blood glucose of injections of carbachol and nor-adrenaline into the lateral hypothalamus of the rat. Note that all injections increased the level of blood glucose but that this increase was greatest with carbachol. No food or water was given during the tests. Data from Coons, Booth, Pitt and Miller; reproduced with permission from Miller (1965).

All of the above studies on drinking behaviour have been conducted in rats. As stated above (§5.1, A) studies with higher mammals have complicated the development of an hypothesis about the central regulation of drinking behaviour. Myers (1964) found that neither cholinergic nor adrenergic stimulation of the cat's lateral or medial hypothalamus elicited drinking, but that injections of ACh, carbachol, nor-adrenaline (NA) or adrenaline (ADR) produced a variety of emotional and autonomic changes. Myers (1964) reported also that drinking was produced by adrenergic stimulation of the VMH of cats, which is not in accord with results obtained by other workers who used rats (see above). In further experiments, Sharpe and Myers (1969) found that NA elicited both eating and drinking when injected into the anterior pre-optic region, LH, or other diencephalic regions of satiated monkeys. ADR, dopamine (DA) and serotonin (5-HT) also produced ingestive responses, but cholinergic substances applied to these same sites did not produce drinking behaviour. Myers (1969) concluded that these very large amounts of ACh or carbachol (1–50 $\mu$g), when injected into the LH of satiated monkeys, blocked food and water intake, but did not elicit eating or drinking. However, NA or 5-HT, also in very large amounts (1–50 $\mu$g), evoked "abnormal" eating and drinking behaviours when injected into the LH in satiated monkeys. Although these experiments with cats and monkeys showed that marked species variations might exist in the central mediation of ingestive behaviours, the very large amounts of substance injected into the brain make their interpretation impossible with regard to normal "physiological" or "biochemical" mechanisms.

It remains unclear whether the data obtained indicate the existence of a cholinergic system for the central mediation of "natural" drinking behaviour. Since administration of anti-cholinergic agents can inhibit completely carbachol-induced drinking, while causing only a slight inhibition of deprivation-induced drinking, it appears that these two types of drinking behaviour are not subserved by identical mechanisms. At present, the cholinergic system does not seem to qualify as a sole substrate for naturally-occurring, thirst-mediated phenomena. Also, there exists an appreciable overlap with regard to function in the diencephalic and limbic areas associated with ingestive behaviours, and stereotaxic methods have not yet been refined to the extent whereby one can discuss, with accuracy, exact implantation sites among various species. Furthermore, the intra-cerebral approach, itself, is of only limited value for monitoring the changes in brain function and behaviour caused by ACh, or other substances, for it cannot be shown whether the applied agents act directly on cellular perikarya and dendrites or on fibre pathways, or on both, and usually very large amounts of test substance have had to be administered to induce behavioural changes (see §5.1 D, below).

### C. Feeding Behaviour

From Grossman's pioneering studies (1960, 1962a, b) it was concluded that food intake in satiated rats was mediated by a central adrenergic mechanism localized mainly in the hypothalamus but which included other brain areas (see also Miller *et al.*, 1964; Fisher and Coury, 1964;

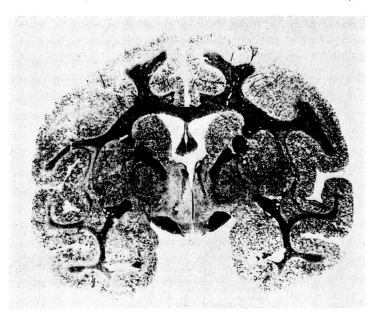

Fig. 5.9. Coronal section of Rhesus monkey brain cut at 24 $\mu$ and stained for cells and fibres by the method of Klüver-Barerra (1953). The tip of the cannula used for intra-hypothalamic injections is in the lateral hypothalamus, dorsal to the optic tract and lateral to the columns of the fornix ($\times 3$) Reproduced with permission from Myers and Sharpe (1968).

Miller, 1965; Slangen and Miller, 1969). Grossman (1964, 1966a) showed further that cholinergic stimulation of the medial septum depressed food intake in hungry rats, and that application of atropine to the VMH did not affect food intake; adrenergic substances (e.g. NA) elicited feeding behaviour. Feeding behaviour has also been elicited by intra-ventricular injections of NA in rats, while carbachol elicited only drinking (Lovett and Singer, 1971). It is now thought that the central "feeding circuit" is much more complex than previously imagined, and the effects of centrally-applied adrenergic and cholinergic agents have differed markedly with regard to the species studied. For example, in rabbits intra-hypothalamic injections of carbachol elicited feeding behaviour (Sommer *et al.*, 1967), while in cats both cholinergic and adrenergic stimulation of similar brain areas caused neither feeding nor drinking behaviour (Myers, 1964). In monkeys, injections of NA into various areas of the diencephalon elicited both feeding and drinking when animals were satiated, while cholinergic agents were ineffective;

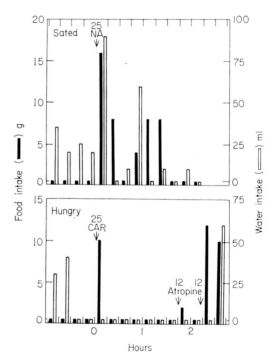

Fig. 5.10. Food and water intake in a Rhesus monkey following injection in to the lateral hypothalamus (at zero hour) of 25 μg nor-adrenaline (*NA*; *top*) or 25 μg carbachol (*CAR*) at the same site two weeks later (*bottom*). Atropine (12 μg) was injected, at arrows, into this same site. Reproduced with permission from Myers (1969).

with hungry and thirsty monkeys, ingestive responses elicited by direct injection into areas such as the lateral hypothalamus were inhibited by cholinergic agents and these effects were prevented by atropine (Myers and Sharpe, 1968; Myers, 1969; Sharpe and Myers, 1969; see Figs 5.9–5.11). It must be concluded that adrenergically-induced feeding behaviour cannot be shown reliably in any species tested, except perhaps for the rat.

## D. *Criticism*

Criticism of the studies performed on ingestive behaviours may help to clarify some of the major problems to be solved by future research. First of all, there has been a definite lack of experimental control with regard to the choice of substances used for intra-cerebral injections. In most studies, cholinergic, anticholinergic, adrenergic and anti-adrenergic substances were tested and NaCl was used to control for

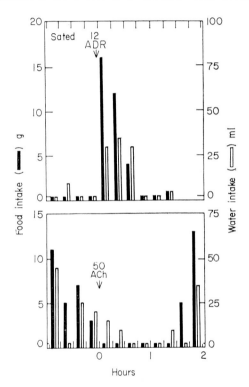

Fɪɢ. 5.11. Effects of adrenaline and ACh on food and water intake in a Rhesus monkey. Adrenaline (ADR) was injected into the lateral hypothalamus at zero hour (*top*), and ACh was injected into the same site two weeks later (*bottom*). Time scale is in hours; 12 and 50 refer to amounts of ADR and ACh injected, in μg. Reproduced with permission from Myers (1969).

volume and osmotic effects (e.g. Grossman, 1960, 1962a). When testing for the possible transmitter mechanisms which govern complex behaviours and which might be associated with changes in the irritability of certain neuronal populations, a variety of known pharmacologically-active substances (e.g. convulsants, anaesthetics, excitatory and inhibitory amino acids) should be used in addition to the substances tested.

Intra-cerebral administration of such agents would evoke or modify feeding and drinking behaviours, as well as other motivated behaviours. Therefore, by using some of these other agents a better understanding of the specificity of both the substances tested and of the behaviours evoked could be gained. For instance, it seems possible that glutamate and GABA, which are, respectively, naturally-occurring excitatory and inhibitory substances of brain, could interfere with feeding and/or drinking behaviour, if applied to certain brain structures. This idea becomes easier to understand when it is considered that intra-hypothalamic injections of both glutamate (Brody *et al.*, 1969) and cholinergic substances (e.g. Bandler, 1969, 1970) have been shown to elicit "attack" behaviour in mammals.

Furthermore, even if peripheral or central injections of atropine do block a response elicited by a cholinergic substance, this does not provide conclusive evidence that the "natural" mechanism for this response is "cholinergic", especially when very large amounts of the cholinergic substance had to be used to elicit the effect. (This same criticism applies to the studies with catecholamines and their antagonists.) Behavioural effects elicited by intra-cerebral injections of large amounts of cholinergic substances and the subsequent blockade of these effects by cholinergic antagonists may simply mean that the cholinergic substances had interacted with cell membranes to change their states of irritability, and that the antagonists had reduced these interactions. It is also conceivable that cholinergic receptors could actually be formed by the brain in response to intra-cerebral injections of large amounts of cholinergic substances; i.e. by processes related to the brain's natural mechanisms of detoxification or desensitization. Even if a given cerebral structure is specific to a given behavioural pattern, it seems likely that the behaviour could be triggered by any one of a variety of chemical substances. Upon further testing of other substances by this method, it is predicted that other transmitter mechanisms will be implicated in the central control of ingestive (and related) behaviours.

Environmental and social influences could also affect the behaviours which may be elicited by the central application of pharmacologically-active substances. In many of the experiments performed on feeding and drinking behaviours, rats were maintained in "individual cages" (e.g. Grossman, 1962a, Myers and Yaksh, 1968; Slangan and Miller, 1969; Levitt *et al.*, 1970; Lovett and Singer, 1971). Also, monkeys are usually housed in "partial isolation", and the experiments cited above were performed while these animals were in restraining chairs (Sharpe and Myers, 1969). Since individual housing (isolation) of mammals causes pronounced changes to occur in emotionality (see e.g. Welch, 1965; Harlow, 1965; Valzelli, 1967; Garattini *et al.*, 1969; Prescott, 1971) and since central cholinergic systems seem to be altered by differential housing (see e.g. Bennett and Rosenzweig, 1971; Essman, 1971, 1972; Table 9), it seems evident that this factor has influenced many of the studies which have been conducted on ingestive behaviours. This criticism becomes even more significant when one considers the extensive anatomical and functional overlap which exists in the central representation of ingestive behaviours and other motivated behaviours. Variations

TABLE 9. Acetylcholine concentration of the cerebral cortex in differentially-housed, drug-treated mice. Reproduced with permission from Essman (1971).

| Housing Condition | Treatment Condition | Mean ($\pm \sigma$) ACh Concentration (n-mol/g) | | | Ratio $\left(\dfrac{\text{"Bound"}}{\text{"Free"}}\right)$ |
|---|---|---|---|---|---|
| | | Whole Tissue ("Total") | Homogenate ("Bound") | Residual ("Free") | |
| Aggregation | Saline | 16·43 (2·30) | 10·00 (1·40) | 6·43 (0·53) | 1·55 |
| | Nicotine | 8·06 (0·49)[a] | 1·22 (0·07)[a] | 6·84 (0·38) | 0·18 |
| Isolation | Saline | 16·00 (1·36) | 4·00 (2·40) | 12·00 (0·32) | 0·33 |
| | Nicotine | 6·87 (0·91)[a] | 3·58 (0·86) | 3·29 (0·36)[a] | 1·09 |

Male CF-1s mice, 25 days of age, were subjected to differential housing for 165 days and then injected intra-peritoneally with 1·0 mg/kg nicotine-$SO_4$ (in 0·9% saline) or with an equivalent volume of 0·9% saline. Forty-five min. after injections, animals were killed and "free" and "bound" fractions of ACh were determined in samples of cerebral cortex.

[a] indicates $p < 0·01$ for comparisons between nicotine-treated $v$ control animals; calculated ratios differed significantly from one another.

in the sizes of test compartments and in the availability of objects in these compartments also could have influenced the results obtained. For example, injection of carbachol into the LH area of rats can produce drinking behaviour, but in the presence of a suitable "attack object" (e.g. a mouse) injection of this same agent into this same area can induce "attack" or "killing" behaviour (e.g. Smith *et al.*, 1970). Hence, the environment of experimental animals, in terms of both their housing conditions and test compartments, should be rigorously controlled. Furthermore, many behavioural patterns and physiological functions of mammals are affected by rhythmically-occurring phenomena (see e.g. Sollberger, 1960, 1965), and this could alter the responses elicited by intra-cerebrally administered cholinergic (or other) substances. A relevant report about the influences of light-dark rhythms on feeding and drinking behaviours in rats has appeared (Zucker, 1971). In this connection, it is noteworthy that the ACh content of brain structures

(Friedman and Walker, 1969, 1972; Hanin *et al.*, 1970; see Fig. 5.12 and Table 10), as well as the levels of other cerebral biogenic amines and their associated enzyme activities (see references in Hanin *et al.*, 1970), also undergo diurnal variation. Diurnal variations in cerebral ACh

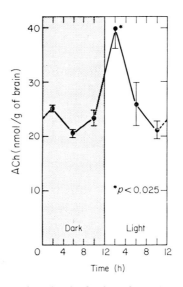

Fig. 5.12. ACh concentrations in the brains of rats killed throughout one 24-hr cycle. Means ± S.E.M. of three or more rats per point; *, indicates that this point of the light phase differed significantly from all other points. Reproduced with permission from Hanin *et al.*, (1970).

TABLE 10. Acetylcholine levels in rat midbrain and caudate nucleus as a function of the time of day. Reproduced with permission from Friedman and Walker (1972).

| Time of day | Midbrain $n$-mol/g ($\pm$S.D.) | Caudate nucleus $n$-mol/g ($\pm$S.D.) |
|---|---|---|
| 6·00 | 32·0 ± 0·7 | 32·7 ± 4·5 |
| 12·00 | 29·5 ± 1·9[c] | 29·2 ± 5·2 |
| 18·00 | 32·1 ± 1·1 | 28·5 ± 3·2 |
| 24·00 | 38·3 ± 1·0[a] | 34·6 ± 4·8[b] |

[a] The difference between maximum and minimum value is statistically significant ($p < 0.01$).
[b] Minimum value significantly different from 24·00 h ($p < 0.05$).
[c] Minimum value significantly different from 6·00 and 18·00 h ($p < 0.05$).
   n = 5 for midbrain; n = 5 pairs for caudate nucleus.

content have been correlated with changes in the toxicities of various cholinergic and anti-cholinergic agents (Friedman and Walker, 1972; Table 11).

Criticisms concerning the routes of injection of test substances also apply to the above studies on ingestive behaviours. As is well known, results obtained with the same drug administered by different routes are subject to much variation and cannot be compared either on a qualitative or on a quantitative basis (see §3.5). With intra-ventricular injections (e.g. Myers and Yaksh, 1968; Lovett and Singer, 1971), test substances enter primarily the CSF compartment but their actions are mediated mainly by their effects on structures lining the ventricles; also, diffusion to the periphery may obscure the exact sites of action of the substances administered (see Rech, 1968). Experiments in which cannulae are used to penetrate the brain for direct injection or implantation of substances (e.g. Grossman, 1960, 1962a) are subject to criticisms based on tissue destruction, pressure effects, diffusional effects, and other effects (see Rech, 1968). Furthermore, with intra-cerebral injections it cannot be determined whether the observed effects are produced by agonistic or blocking actions of the test substance, or whether mechanical and/or pharmacological interference with excitatory or inhibitory pathways play significant roles (e.g. Izquierdo and Izquierdo, 1971). Iontophoretic methods are subject to many of the criticisms outlined above for cannulae, and in addition, do not permit study of whole populations of cells which necessarily represent complex behaviours.

## 5.2 Emotion and Motivated Behaviours

### A. Introduction

Since an emotion can be defined as a component of motivation, it is not possible to discuss separately the central factors which govern emotion and motivation. Hence, it will be assumed that many neural functions are common to emotional and motivated behaviours, and that these behaviours are necessary requirements for learning and memory. It may be considered that emotionality and motivation are associated with adjusting the level of behavioural arousal in the animal and that this adjustment affects processes of learning and memory (see Hebb, 1955, 1958; Fig. 2.7). Klüver and Bucy (1937) and Papez (1937) first localized "emotions" in the telencephalon, but it is now known that many other, if not all, brain areas are associated with emotion, as well as with motivation and complex behaviours. With regard to emotion and motivation, the most widely studied structures have been hypothalamus, septum, other diencephalic and limbic structures and the reticular formation. The importance of diencephalic and limbic

TABLE 11. Circadian $LD_{50}$ values for cholinergic compounds in mice. Reproduced with permission from Friedman and Walker (1972).

| Agent | $LD_{50}$ values—mg/kg (i.p.) Time of day (h) | | | |
| --- | --- | --- | --- | --- |
| | 6.00 | 12.00 | 18.00 | 24.00 |
| Cholinomimetic | | | | |
| Acetylcholine Cl | 168·70 ± 21·40 | 195·90 ± 13·60[b] | 185·80 ± 15·20 | 162·20 ± 13·70 |
| Carbachol Cl | 0·37 ± 0·06 | 0·56 ± 0·08[b] | 0·40 ± 0·10 | 0·56 ± 0·07 |
| Pilocarpine HCl | 154·50 ± 15·30 | 179·40 ± 8·20 | 181·10 ± 7·10[a] | 158·50 ± 9·70 |
| Oxotremorine | 3·20 ± 0·20 | 4·10 ± 0·97[a] | 3·80 ± 0·10 | 3·00 ± 0·20 |
| Anti-cholinesterase | | | | |
| Eserine. $SO_4$ | 0·71 ± 0·05[b] | 0·63 ± 0·03 | 0·59 ± 0·01 | 0·51 ± 0·05 |
| Neostigmine. $CH_3SO_4$ | 0·23 ± 0·06 | 0·28 ± 0·03 | 0·36 ± 0·05[b] | 0·29 ± 0·03 |
| Anti-cholinergic | | | | |
| Atropine $SO_4$ | 243·20 ± 7·60 | 191·50 ± 28·80 | 223·90 ± 9·50 | 243·90 ± 21·40 |
| Scopolamine HCl (i.v.) | 118·40 ± 5·50 | 104·40 ± 15·03 | 133·70 ± 15·85[a] | 117·60 ± 8·20 |
| Atropine $CH_3NO_3$ (i.v.) | 9·18 ± 0·48 | 8·67 ± 0·76 | 9·78 ± 0·76[b] | 9·47 ± 1·76 |
| Cholinomimetic | | | | |
| Acetylcholine Cl (After Atropine $CH_3NO_3$, 25 mg/kg, i.p.) | 180·70 ± 19·80 | 223·90 ± 15·50 | 230·70 ± 9·20[b] | 187·90 ± 40·00 |
| Eserine $SO_4$ | 1·00 ± 0·03 | 1·01 ± 0·02[a] | 0·97 ± 0·03 | 0·86 ± 0·09 |

All values represent means ± standard deviations.
[a] Difference between maximum and minimum values significant at $p < 0.05$.
[b] Difference between maximum and minimum values significant at $p < 0.01$. n = 9–11 mice/dose.

structures as major anatomical substrates for emotional (affective) components of behaviour has been long realized (see e.g. reviews by MacLean 1949; Fulton, 1951, Fig. 5.1), and this concept has been supported by the results of many studies in which these cerebral areas have been electrically stimulated (see e.g. Hess, 1949, 1957; MacLean and Delgado, 1953; MacLean, 1957). Throughout this anatomical system are located "pleasure centres" (especially in septum and pre-optic region of hypothalamus) and "punishment centres" (especially in amygdala, hypothalamus, midbrain tegmentum and thalamus; Olds, 1958).

In reviewing experimental evidence based mainly on EEG data, Lindsley (1951, 1957) proposed that the thalamic and brain stem reticular formation may be of prime significance in the regulation of "non-specific motivational processes". Hence, it is evident, even at the anatomical level, that emotional and motivational processes are intimately related to the arousal system (see Chapter 2; Zanchetti, 1967; Fig. 5.13). Due to the extensive overlap of mechanisms for arousal, emotionality, and motivational behaviour in the reticular formation, it seems quite unlikely that separate anatomical or functional entities can be shown for these systems. Perhaps it is best to assume that the balance between the levels of arousal and emotionality may govern the level of motivation in an organism as well as its potential for learning and memory. Undoubtedly, many of the processes underlying these complex functions are cholinergic, and some investigators believe that by using techniques of intra-cerebral injection, areas of the brain may be "coded" pharmacologically with regard to functional specificity (e.g. Grossman, 1960, 1962a; Fisher and Coury, 1962; Miller, 1965). Although it is most unlikely that discrete anatomical pathways for arousal, emotionality and motivation will ever be shown by this method, these studies have shed some light on the association of cholinergic mechanisms with higher central functions.

MacLean and Delgado (1953) have shown that injections of ACh into the rostral part of the hippocampus produced marked affective reactions in the cat and that pinching of the animal's tail in these cases could produce a form of "attack" behaviour. Similar emotional-affective responses, related to "fear and escape" ("rage"), have been produced by intra-ventricular (e.g. Feldberg and Sherwood, 1954; Feldberg and Malcolm, 1959; Feldberg and Fleischauer, 1962, 1963, 1965), or by intra-hypothalamic (Decsi and Várszegi, 1969) injection of *d*-tubocurarine (*d*-TC) in mammals. Clear-cut rage reactions have also been elicited by direct injections of carbachol into the anteromedial hypothalamus of cats, or by electrical stimulation of this region (Baxter, 1966; Várszegi and Decsi, 1967). An analysis of the many types of emotional-affective responses which can be elicited by intra-cerebral

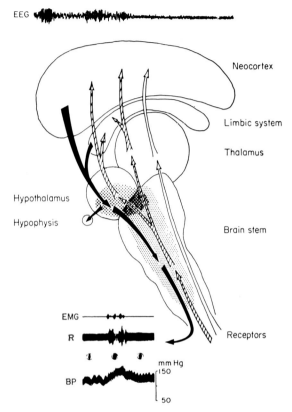

Fɪɢ. 5.13. Roles of the brain stem reticular formation in the mediation of emotional experience and emotional expression. Peripheral receptors, through specific sensory pathways (*white arrows*), influence specific thalamic nuclei and specific sensory areas of the cortex; these pathways are essential in sensory perception, but not in emotion. Peripheral receptors also influence the brain stem reticular formation (*stippled area*) and these ascending retiular influences (*striped arrows*) act upon the neocortex and limbic system to elicit arousal (see EEG at top of the figure) which is thought to be necessary for emotional experience. Reticular influences may also act on mesodiencephalic mechanisms to elicit "rage" (*cross-hatched area*). The expression of rage occurs via descending reticular pathways (*black arrows*), and consists of both somatic and visceral phenomena, as indicated in the lower left of the figure, by increases in muscular activity, respiration, and blood pressure and by pupillary dilatation. Other ascending and descending inter-relationships are indicated. Reproduced with permission from Zanchetti (1967).

injections of cholinomimetic and cholinolytic agents into various cerebral structures of the cat has been presented (Rech, 1968; see Table 12 and Fig. 5.14).

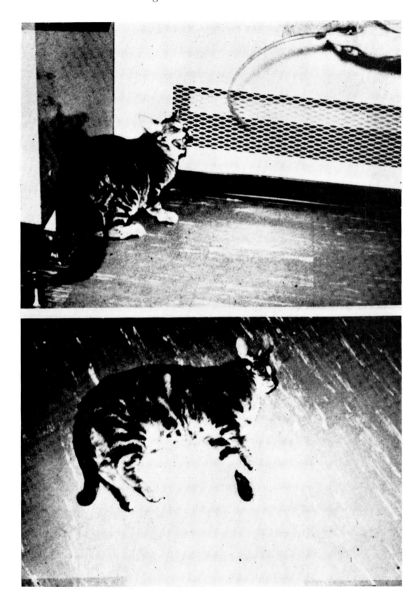

FIG. 5.14. *Top:* Cholinergic stimulation (10 μg carbachol) of the lateral hypo-thalamus of a cat. Note pupillary dilatation, piloerection, hissing and "fear-like" withdrawal to piece of tubing. Hissing and spitting behaviours accompanied the even-tual attack of the tubing. *Bottom:* Adrenergic stimulation of the same site, with 10 μg adrenaline, caused pupillary constriction, proneness and absence of emotional behaviour. Reproduced with permission from Myers (1964).

TABLE 12. Some effects of intra-cerebrally-administered cholinergic agents on physiology and behaviour

| Agent | Site of injection (or implantation) | Species | Effect | Reference |
|---|---|---|---|---|
| ACh | H, V | cat | sleep-like states | Dikshit (1934c, 1935) |
| | H | cat, dog | effects on blood pressure, heart rate and respiration | Dikshit (1934b); Chang et al. (1937a, 1938a) |
| | V | human | thermoregulatory response | Henderson and Wilson (1936) |
| | SON | dog | inhibited water-induced diuresis | Pickford (1947); Duke et al. (1950) |
| | Hip | cat | emotional-affective responses; attack | MacLean and Delgado (1953) |
| | LH | rat | polydipsia in sated subjects | Grossman (1960) |
| | PO, IPN, MMT, MFB | cat | sleep | Hernández-Peón et al. (1963a); |
| | S, PO, Cau | cat | rage reaction | Hernández-Peón et al. (1963a) Velluti and Hernández-Peón (1963) |
| | CiG | monkey | bursts of EEG hypersynchrony | Delgado (1966) |
| | GP | rat | elicited rest tremor | Ruždik and Stern (1966) |
| | Am | cat | aggressiveness, seizures, behavioural inhibition, sleep | Allikmets et al. (1969) |
| | Am, Hip | monkey | EEG seizure activity | Delgado and DeFeudis (1969) |
| | V | rat | increased colonic temperature | Myers and Yaksh (1968) |
| | PO/AH | rat | immediate decrease in body and hypothalamic temperature | Beckman and Carlisle (1969); Kirkpatrick and Lomax (1970); Crawshaw (1973) |
| Carbachol | LH | rat | polydipsia in sated subjects | Grossman (1960) |
| | Cau | cat | elicited contralateral circling | Stevens et al. (1961) |
| | DPH | rabbit | impaired aversive CR; facilitated appetitive CR | Kalyuzhnyi (1962) |
| | S, MRF | cat | alertness (low dose); rage reaction (high dose) | Hernández-Peón et al. (1963a) |
| | LH | rat | convulsions (high doses) | Miller et al. (1964) |

TABLE 12—contd.

| Agent | Site of injection (or implantation) | Species | Effect | Reference |
|---|---|---|---|---|
| Carbachol—(contd.) | S | rat | polydipsia in sated subjects; impaired aversive CR; prevented acquisition of CR | Grossman (1964) |
| | AH, PH, LH | cat | attack; pupillary dilatation; twitching | Myers (1964) |
| | LH, MRF | cat | contralateral circling; increased heart rate | Myers (1964) |
| | MiTN, RTN | rat | impaired acquisition of aversive CR | Grossman et al. (1965) |
| | LH | rat | elicited polydipsia; stimulated renal reabsorption of water; increased blood glucose level | Miller (1965) |
| | MRF | rat | impaired acquisition of CR | Grossman and Grossman (1966) |
| | MRF | rat | initial stimulation: loss of aversive CR and escape; repeated stimulation: facilitated aversive CR | Grossman (1966b) |
| | PO | rat | elicited polydipsia | Quartermain and Miller (1966) |
| | Cau | cat | elicited tremor | Baxter et al. (1966a, 1967a); Connor et al. (1967) |
| | AH | cat | rage reaction | Baxter (1966); Várszegi and Decsi (1967) |
| | Cau, VL | cat | impaired appetitive CR (low dose) | Hull et al. (1967) |
| | Cau, SubT | cat | elicited rage and hyperthermia (high dose) | Hull et al. (1967) |
| | H | rabbit | elicited feeding behaviour | Sommer et al. (1967) |
| | MRF | rat | facilitated aversive CR with low shock; impaired behaviour in high shock situation | Grossman (1968) |
| | Hip | cat | localized seizure discharges | Baker and Benedict (1968a) |
| | S | rat | elicited polydipsia; increased activity in open field | Greene (1968) |
| | AH, VMH | rat | elicited polydipsia in sated subjects | Hendler and Blake (1969) |
| | V | rat | elicited changes in blood pressure | Brezenoff and Jenden (1969, 1970) |
| | LH | monkey | prevented food and water intake in sated subjects | Sharpe and Myers (1969) |
| | AH, LH | rat | facilitated attack and killing | Bandler (1969); Smith et al. (1970) |

TABLE 12—*contd.*

| Agent | Site of injection (or implantation) | Species | Effect | Reference |
|---|---|---|---|---|
| Carbachol— (*contd.*) | Hip | rat | decreased learning of an alternation task | Greene and Lomax (1970) |
| | PO | rat | increased colonic temperature | Avery (1970, 1971) |
| | S, LH, AT MiTN, MTN, VMT | rat | elicited polydipsia in sated subjects | Krikstone and Levitt (1970) |
| | V | rat | facilitated attack and killing | Bandler (1971a, b) |
| | Am | rat | elicited drinking in sated and deprived subjects | Lovett and Singer (1971) |
| | | rat | EEG and behavioural seizures; impaired acquisition of aversive CR | Belluzzi (1972) |
| | VMH, PH | rat | increased blood pressure and heart rate | Brezenoff (1972) |
| | DMH, PMH | rat | decreased blood pressure and heart rate | Brezenoff (1972) |
| DFP | SON | dog | decreased water-induced diuresis | Duke *et al.* (1950) |
| | Cau | rabbit | contralateral circling | White (1956) |
| | SON | dog | increased spontaneous uterine activity | Abrahams and Pickford (1956) |
| | Hip | cat | localized seizures | Baker and Benedict (1967b) |
| | PO | rat | elicited polydipsia in sated subjects | Winson and Miller (1970) |
| | Cau | cat | elicited rest tremor | Lalley *et al.* (1970) |
| eserine | SON | dog | decreased water-induced diuresis | Pickford (1947) |
| | SON | dog | increased spontaneous uterine activity | Abrahams and Pickford (1956) |
| | Cau | cat | elicited test tremor | Baker *et al.* (1967a); Lalley *et al.* (1970) |
| | PO | rat | elicited drinking in sated subjects | Miller and Chien (1968); Winson and Miller (1970) |
| | S, AT, PO, LH | rat | elicited drinking in sated subjects | Levitt and Boley (1970) |
| | PH | rat | increased blood pressure and heart rate | Brezenoff (1972) |
| | Am | rat | produced deficit in acquisition of aversive CR | Belluzzi (1972) |

TABLE 12—*contd.*

| Agent | Site of injection (or implantation) | Species | Effect | Reference |
|---|---|---|---|---|
| atropine | PO, IPN, MMT | cat | blocked ACh-induced sleep; elicited alertness | Velluti and Hernández-Peón (1963) |
| | VMH | rat | impaired appetitive CR; facilitated aversive CR | Grossman (1966a) |
| | S, AH, LH | rat | antagonized carbachol-induced drinking | Levitt and Fisher (1966, 1967) |
| | MiTN | rat | facilitated aversive and appetitive CR | Grossman and Peters (1966) |
| | RTN | rat | impaired acquisition of aversive and appetitive CR's | Grossman and Peters (1966) |
| | Hip | rat | impaired appetitive CR | Khavari and Maickel (1967) |
| | Cau, SubT | cat | antagonized carbachol effects | Hull et al. (1967) |
| | S | cat | produced deficit in aversive CR | Hamilton et al. (1968). |
| | S, AT | rat | antagonized carbachol-induced drinking | Levitt (1970) |
| | MiTN, MTN | rat | suppressed attack and killing | Bandler (1971a) |
| | Cau-Put, GP | rat | elicited contralateral circling | Costall et al. (1972) |
| scopolamine | Hip | cat | antagonized localized seizure activity | Baker and Benedict (1968, 1970) |
| | Cau | cat | antagonized rest tremor induced by cholinomimetics and anti-ChE agents | Lalley et al. (1970) |
| d-TC | V | cat | tremor-like responses; restlessness; motor seizures | Feldberg and Sherwood (1954); Feldberg and Malcolm (1959); Feldberg and Fleischauer (1962, 1963, 1965) |
| | MRF | cat | motor seizures | Kumagai et al. (1962) |
| | Hip | cat | high voltage EEG spiking | Endröczi et al. (1963) |
| | Cc | mouse | tremors; motor seizures | Molnár et al. (1967) |
| | Hip | cat | localized seizure activity | Baker et al. (1965); Baker and Benedict (1967, 1970) |

TABLE 12—contd.

| Agent | Site of injection (or implantation) | Species | Effect | Reference |
|---|---|---|---|---|
| d-TC—(contd.) | H | cat | pressor response | Fletcher and Pradhan (1969) |
| | AH | cat | "fear and escape" reaction | Decsi and Várszegi (1969) |
| oxotremorine (or tremorine) | Cau, GP | rat | elicited rest tremor | Blažević et al. (1965); Cox and Potkonjak (1969) |
| | H | rat | elicited hypotensive responses | Brezenoff and Wirecki (1970) |
| HC-3 | GP | rat | prevented against rest tremor | Ruždik (1965) |
| | V | dog | produced amygdaloid spiking and blocked hippocampal theta activity | Domino (1966); Domino et al. (1967, 1968) |

Abbreviations:

AH, anterior hypothalamus
Am, amygdaloid complex
AT, anterior thalamus
Cau, caudate nucleus
Cc, cerebral cortex
CiG, cingulate gyrus
CR, conditioned response
DMH, dorso-medial hypothalamus
DPH, dorso-posterior hypothalamus
GP, globus pallidus
H, hypothalamus (various regions)
Hip, hippocampus
IPN, interpenduncular nucleus
LH, lateral hypothalamus
MFB, medial forebrain bundle
MiTN, midline thalamic nuclei

MMT, medial midbrain tegmentum
MRF, mesencephalic reticular formation
MTN, medial thalamic nuclei
PH, posterior hypothalamus
PMH, pre-mammillary hypothalamus
PO, pre-optic region of hypothalamus
Put, putamen
RTN, reticular thalamic nuclei
S, septal area
SON, supraoptic nucleus of hypothalamus
SubT, subthalamus
V, cerebral ventricles
VL, ventro-lateral thalamic nucleus
VMH, ventro-medial hypothalamus
VMT, ventral midbrain tegmentum

## B. *Attack Behaviour*

"Attack behaviour" may be considered to be a component of both the "affective-defence" ("rage") reaction and of "predatory aggression". The cerebral areas associated with the emotional and the goal-directed components of attack behaviour, though appearing to be closely linked, may be anatomically distinct (Moyer, 1968). Attack behaviours have been associated with the lateral hypothalamus (e.g. see references in Bandler, 1970), certain limbic structures (e.g. MacLean and Delgado, 1953), the ventral midbrain tegmentum (Bandler *et al.*, 1972) and regions of the thalamus (e.g. Bandler, 1971a). Integration of the several autonomic and somatic components of attack behaviour may occur in the hypothalamus (e.g. Hess and Brugger, 1943, Hunsperger, 1956, Wasman and Flynn, 1962). Continued interest in the study of attack behaviours has stemmed mainly from their use as model systems for human aggression.

Predatory aggression (e.g. frog- or mouse-killing by rats; rat-killing by cats) has been the most widely studied type of attack behaviour. This behaviour is stereotyped and stimulus-specific (e.g. Karli, 1956; Wasman and Flynn, 1962), and is characterized by a lack of affective display and by a "biting" form of attack directed at the neck region of the prey. This type of response is heavily dependent upon the presence of a suitable "attack object" (e.g. Levinson and Flynn, 1965; MacDonnell and Flynn, 1966a, b). Direct injections of carbachol, ACh-plus-eserine, or neostigmine into sites of the lateral hypothalamus (LH) facilitated frog and mouse-killing responses in natural "killer" rats at sites which seemed to be distinct from those regulating drinking behaviour (Bandler, 1969, 1970; Smith *et al.*, 1970). Since systemically-administered atropine, but not direct injections of atropine, into "attack" sites, inhibited attack behaviour in Bandler's experiments, it was suggested that attack behaviour might be diffusely represented in the brain. In further studies, it was shown that direct injections of carbachol into sites of the medial and midline thalamus (Bandler, 1971a) or ventral midbrain tegmentum (Bandler, 1971b) also facilitated attack and killing behaviours in rats. However, in these studies, injection of atropine into the same sites usually blocked the effects of carbachol. It was shown further that concurrent application of atropine to thalamic sites and carbachol to hypothalamic sites prevented the facilitatory effect of carbachol on attack and killing behaviours (see Table 13). Lesions to the septal area have also been shown to cause increased aggressiveness (e.g. Wheatley, 1944; Brady and Nauta, 1953; King, 1958) and mouse-killing in rats (Karli, 1956), and direct cholinergic stimulation of the septal area can elicit rage in the cat (Hernández-Peón, 1965). Direct injections of amitone (an anti-ChE agent) into the septum increased aggressiveness and mouse-killing in rats by an atropine-sensitive mechanism (Igić *et al.*, 1970).

Although the above evidence indicates that cholinergic mechanisms may play a significant role in the mediation of attack behaviour, further experimental control is necessary. In this regard, Bandler (1971a) reported that intra-thalamic injections of NA, 5-HT, strychnine and dibenzyline did not alter consistently the aggressive behaviour of rats,

TABLE 13. Mean latencies of attack and kill for blockade by atropine at dorsomedial thalamus of hypothalamically-facilitated predatory aggression[a]. Reproduced with permission from Bandler (1971a).

| Site | Attack latency (s) | | | Kill latency (s) | | |
|------|------|------|----------|------|------|----------|
|      | Ct-H | Ca-H | Ca-H/At-T | Ct-H | Ca-H | Ca-H/At-T |
| 2R   | 82·2  | 3·3[b]   | 177·5 | 139·7 | 6·3[c]   | 194·0 |
| 12R  | 146·8 | 9·0[c]   | 118·8 | 263·9 | 25·8[c]  | 197·3 |
| 18R  | 137·3 | 108·0    | 235·7 | 216·8 | 131·0[b] | 269·3 |
| 18L  | 197·2 | 67·7[d]  | 177·0 | 253·2 | 149·0[c] | 219·0 |
| 26R  | 262·5 | 34·0[c]  | 146·0 | 300·0 | 45·0[c]  | 328·0 |
| 26L  | 253·0 | 31·0[d]  | 118·3 | 274·0 | 83·0[c]  | 199·0 |
| 37R  | 281·0 | 46·0[c]  | 244·0 | 305·0 | 55·0[c]  | 252·0 |
| 37L  | 244·0 | 35·0[d]  | 247·2 | 262·0 | 40·0[c]  | 286·0 |

Abbreviations: Ca, carbachol stimulation; At, atropine stimulation; Ct, control stimulation; H, hypothalamus; T, thalamus. All comparisons are with the control (Ct) condition; R and L signify the right and left hypothalamic implants.

[a] All *t*-tests (two-tailed) on 4 df.
[b] $p < 0.05$.
[c] $p < 0.01$.
[d] $p < 0.001$.

Note that application of atropine at thalamic sites prevented carbachol-induced facilitation of aggressiveness at hypothalamic sites.

but he provided no data for this. However, it has been shown that intra-hypothalamic injections of glutamate, a potent CNS stimulant and possible excitatory neurotransmitter, can elicit directed attack behaviour in cats which is similar to that elicited by cholinergic agents (Brody *et al.*, 1969). The findings that systemically-injected imipramine exerted a blocking action on electrically-elicited hypothalamic attack in cats and that this mechanism was not affected by atropine indicated further that the "attack" mechanism may not be exclusively cholinergic (Dubinsky and Goldberg, 1971). These studies, taken together with the recent findings that intra-hypothalamic injections of chlorpromazine (an adrenergic blocking agent) caused aggressiveness and attack in rats (Leibowitz and Miller, 1969) and that NA facilitated aggressiveness and attack when injected into ventral midbrain tegmental areas (Bandler, 1971b), indicate that adrenergic mechanisms may also play significant roles in the central mediation of aggressive behaviour (see e.g. review by Reis, 1971).

### 5.3 Other Emotional-Motivational Behaviours; Learning and Memory

#### A. Introduction

It has been suggested that central cholinergic systems may be involved in the mediation of, and in the selective inhibition of responding (e.g.

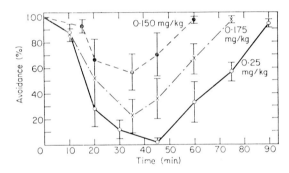

Fig. 5.15. Effects of eserine on conditioned pole-jumping behaviour in rats. The mean avoidance behaviour ($\pm$S.E.M.) for each group of six animals at three doses of eserine is given at various time intervals after injection. Per cent avoidance is given per block of ten trials at the times indicated. N-methyl-atropine (2·1 mg/kg, s.c.) was administered 30 min. prior to eserine salicylate (s.c.). With the 0·25 mg/kg dose of eserine, it was shown that increases in brain ACh content and concurrent inhibition of brain AChE activity coincided temporally with the period of avoidance depression. Reproduced with permission from Rosecrans *et al.*, (1968).

McCleary, 1961, 1966; Russell *et al.*, 1961; Carlton, 1963, 1969; Leaf and Muller, 1966; Reeves, 1966; Stein, 1969; Russell, 1969), and hence, in operant behaviours (e.g. Pfeiffer and Jenny, 1957; Stark and Boyd, 1963; Goldberg *et al.*, 1963, 1965) and in memory coding (e.g. Deutsch, 1966, 1969; Rosenzweig *et al.*, 1967). Most behaviours, whether positively or negatively motivated, can be depressed by systemic administration of cholinergic agonists (see e.g. Goldberg *et al.*, 1963, 1965; Jung and Boyd, 1966; Vaillant, 1967; Khavari, 1971; see also references

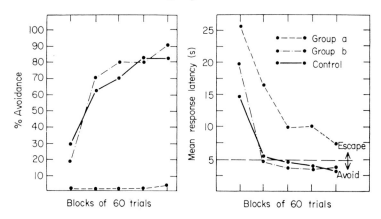

FIG. 5.16. Acquisition of a shuttle-box (escape) avoidance response by rats receiving crystalline carbachol (0·5–5 μg) in the medial septal area (Group *a*), or in an area immediately below the medial septal area (Group *b*), and by rats which were operated upon but not given the drug (Control). Note that application of carbachol to the medial septal area (5 min. before daily training sessions) impaired acquisition of these responses. Reproduced with permission from Grossman (1964).

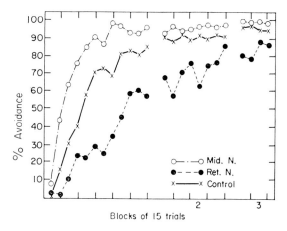

FIG. 5.17. Acquisition and performance of a shuttle-box avoidance response following central application of atropine (1–2 μg crystalline implant) or sham stimulation in rats. Note that atropine application to the dorsolateral thalamus at the level of the reticular nuclei (*Ret. N.*) impaired performance while its application to midline nuclei (*Mid. N*) facilitated this behaviour. Reproduced with permission from Grossman and Peters (1966).

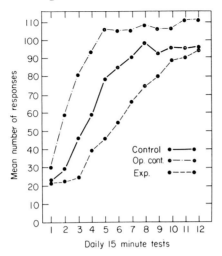

FIG. 5.18. Facilitation by implant-produced lesions (Op. cont.) and impairment by cholinergic stimulation (Exp.), of the same site in the MRF, of acquisition of a bar pressing habit (appetitive behaviour) in rats. Acquisition of bar-pressing is shown beginning with the first session during which each rat met a minimal criterion of 10 responses/15 minutes. For cholinergic stimulation, carbachol was applied 5 min. before each 15-min. test. Reproduced with permission from Grossman and Grossman (1966).

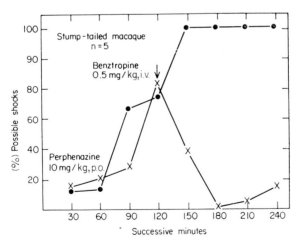

FIG. 5.19. Benztropine reversal of the anti-avoidance effect of perphenazine in a group of five stump-tailed macaques. Perphenazine (10 mg/kg, p.o.) was administered at the start of each session; *arrow* indicates the time of benztropine injection. Perphenazine alone (●—●) caused complete loss of avoidance lever pressing 150 min. after start of the session; injection of benztropine at the 120th minute produced complete restoration of normal responding by the 180th minute of the session (×—×). Reproduced with permission from Hanson *et al.*, (1970).

above). Evidence that the behavioural effects of systemically-administered anti-ChE agents may be of central origin has been provided by
the demonstration that the induced behavioural changes can be related
temporally to decreases in cerebral AChE activity and to increases in
cerebral ACh content (e.g. Goldberg *et al.*, 1963; Rosecrans *et al.*, 1968;
Domino and Olds, 1968; Figs. 5.15, 5.20). Also, it has been shown that
the effects of atropine and scopolamine on learned behaviour were

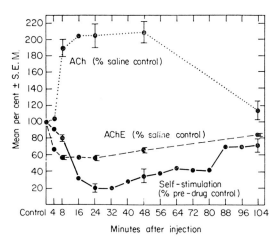

FIG. 5.20. Correlation of self-stimulation behaviour, brain ACh content and brain
AChE activity after injections of eserine (100 μg/kg, s.c.) into rats. Mean per cent
(± S.E.M.) of control animals. Each point represents the mean of at least 6 animals.
Note that the increase in brain ACh, the decrease in brain AChE, and the depression
of self-stimulation are correlated, but that the changes in ACh and AChE preceded the
behavioural alterations. Reproduced with permission from Domino and Olds (1968).

analogous when intra-peritoneal and intra-ventricular routes of injection
were compared (Khavari, 1971).

Conditioned avoidance responses require negative reinforcement,
and hence can serve as learning models (see Skinner, 1953). Since
centrally-active cholinomimetic and cholinolytic agents affect these
responses, a means has been provided for examining cholinergic
mechanisms in relation to motivation and learning. In general, lesions
or direct cholinergic stimulation (e.g. with carbachol) of septal or
hippocampal areas (Fig. 5.1) cause impairment of avoidance responses
while directly-applied cholinergic antagonists generally improve performance (see e.g. Grossman, 1964; Racine and Kimble, 1965; Greene
and Lomax, 1970; references above, and Fig. 5.16).

It is generally believed that both learning and memory involve long-
lasting alterations in synaptic transmission (see e.g. Hebb, 1949; Kandel

and Spencer, 1968; Rosenzweig *et al.*, 1972) and that drugs which affect synaptic transmission should affect information storage and retrieval (see Glassman, 1969). Recent evidence has indicated further that the morphology of the brain, in particular that of axons and dendrites, might undergo change in response to learning and experience (see §5.4, below). Deutsch (1966) has suggested that increased learning promotes an increase in the production of neurotransmitter, but that learning is not due to an increase in the numbers of neurones responding to behavioural input. Other workers (see e.g. John, 1967) have maintained a rather opposite view. On a more molar level, behavioural performance appears to be determined in part by the level of arousal of the animal. This concept has given rise to an arousal or "activation" theory of emotion and motivation (e.g. see Lindsley, 1951; Schlosberg, 1954; Hebb, 1955; Fig. 2.7) and hence to the involvement of the reticular-activating system in processes of motivation and learning.

### B. *Roles of the Septum and Hippocampus*

From studies based on AChE staining and ChAc activities, it has been suggested that a "cholinergic limbic system" either arises from, or traverses, the septal area and innervates the hippocampus (see e.g. Lewis and Shute, 1967, Lewis *et al.*, 1967; Shute and Lewis, 1967; Girgis, 1973; see Figs 2.15–2.18) and the cerebral cortex (Krnjević and Silver, 1965; Figs 2.4, 2.18). Also, electrical stimulation of the septal area of cats has been shown to increase cortical ACh release (Szerb, 1967; Fig. 6.10), and septal lesions can reduce or abolish cortical ACh release produced by administration of amphetamine or scopolamine (Nistri *et al.*, 1972; Pepeu, 1972; see Chapter 6). Further evidence supporting a role for the septum in the cholinergic mediation of function in higher brain centres is derived from the findings that: (1) after its destruction in rats, brain ACh content is decreased, particularly in the cerebral cortex (Pepeu *et al.*, 1971, 1973); and (2) septal lesions have been shown to affect emotionality, locomotor activity, motivation and learning (e.g. Brady and Nauta, 1953; McCleary, 1961; Mulas and Pepeu, 1970; Fried, 1972). However, it should be noted that the septum is also rich in catecholaminergic elements (e.g. Fuxe *et al.*, 1969), and therefore, that its complex functions may well be mediated by an interplay between cholinergic and nor-adrenergic, and possibly other, mechanisms.

It is believed that the septal area is an important relay station in the central regulation of motivated behaviours. Septal lesions can produce a decrement in the strength of conditioned emotional responses in animals, even though they appear more "emotional" than controls (Brady and Nauta, 1953). Septal lesions have been shown to impair passive avoidance behaviour (i.e. avoidance behaviour in situations in which a specific response must be withheld to avoid electric shock), but to improve learning in active avoidance situations (e.g. King, 1958; McCleary, 1961; Meyers, 1965; Fried, 1972; Albert and Mah, 1973). It is noteworthy that pathways project from both the septal area and amygdala to the reticular-activating system, and that lesions of the amygdala can prevent the behavioural effects (e.g. increased aggressiveness) caused by septal lesions (King, 1958). This seems to indicate quite clearly that increased arousal is necessary for the generation of emotional behaviours (see Fig. 5.13). Rates of self-stimulation produced at specific sites in the septal area correlate well with food or water deprivation (Brady *et al.*, 1957; Olds, 1958). Thus, the septal area appears to contain mechanisms which are associated with the regulation of many of the organism's basic drives (e.g. Grossman, 1964), and hence, with "survival of the species" (MacLean, 1958; see Fig. 5.1).

It has been long known that the hippocampus may be concerned with "recent memory" and learning (e.g. von Bechterew, 1900; Glees and Griffith, 1952; Scoville and Milner, 1957; Penfield and Milner, 1958; Victor *et al.*, 1961) in humans. Other suggested functions for the hippocampus include: (1) a role in seizure activity (e.g. Greene and Shimamoto, 1953; MacLean, 1957; see § 3.3); (2) a role in emotional reactions (see §5.2); (3) a role in the regulation of reticular activation of other regions of the cerebral cortex; and (4) an involvement with certain visceral activities (see e.g. Papez, 1937; Greene, 1960; Meissner, 1966).

As a result of the findings outlined above, intensive study has been undertaken on the behavioural effects produced by the application of cholinergic agents to the septum and amygdala-hippocampus regions. Grossman (1964) showed that cholinergic stimulation of the medial septal region of rats altered a number of motivational systems. Among the effects shown were: (1) elicitation of drinking in satiated animals and increasing of water intake in thirsty animals (see §5.1); (2) impairment of acquisition of escape-avoidance responses and of performance of previously-acquired avoidance behaviour (see Fig. 5.16). In further studies, it was shown that application of atropine to the septal area of cats (like septal lesions) caused a deficit in passive avoidance (Hamilton *et al.*, 1968, 1970). Green (1968) showed that implantation of crystalline carbachol into the medial septal region of rats increased their activity in an open field, but no evidence indicated that these animals became more "fearful". These results lend support to the hypothesis that cholinergic mechanisms in the septal area may be involved in mediating the response inhibition and changes in motor activity which are concerned with motivational processes.

The septal nuclei, like the lateral pre-optic region and hypothalamus, seem to be implicated in the integration of limbic system functions, since the major pathways connecting the thalamic and brain stem reticular formation with the hippocampus and amygdala merge in this region. Several studies have indicated that the hippocampus receives a cholinergic input from the medial septal nucleus and the nucleus of the diagonal band (e.g. Lewis and Shute, 1967; Lewis *et al.*, 1967; McGeer *et al.*, 1969; Fonnum, 1970), and "chronic" lesions to the medial septum prevent cholinergic input to the hippocampus and cause decreases in its ACh and choline contents and ChAc activity (Kuhar *et al.*, 1973). In other experiments, Sethy *et al.*, (1973) have shown that "acute" lesions to the medial septal area in rats caused a significant increase in the ACh content of hippocampus during the first 16 hr after the lesion. Also, the AChE activity of the hippocampus is markedly reduced by transection of the fimbria (Shute and Lewis, 1961; Storm-Mathisen, 1970; Table 14).

TABLE 14. Loss of AChE from hippocampus after interruption of fimbria. Reproduced with permission from Storm-Mathisen (1970).

| Rat | Survival time (days) | Activities in $\mu$mol/min./g dry wt.[a] | | | | Relative activities | |
|---|---|---|---|---|---|---|---|
| | | Normal side | | Operated side | | Normal | Operated |
| | | P | R | P | R | P/R | P/R |
| L-2 | $4\frac{1}{2}$ | 59·4 ± 6·9 (5) | 27·7 ± 1·3 (4) | 14·4 ± 0·5 (5) | 9·5 ± 0·5 (6) | 2·2 | 1·5 |
| L-4 | $4\frac{1}{2}$ | 74·8 ± 7·8 (5) | 42·3 ± 6·4 (5) | 9·7 ± 0·7 (6) | 9·3 ± 1·1 (5) | 1·8 | 1·0 |
| L-7 | 7 | 54·5 ± 3·9 (6) | 26·2 ± 5·8 (4) | 10·5 ± 1·2 (6) | 6·8 ± 0·6 (5) | 2·1 | 1·5 |

[a] Assayed by radiochemical method (Fonnum (1969a,b); mean values ± S.E.M.; numbers of samples in brackets.

Symbols: P, 80–100 $\mu$m wide samples containing stratum pyramidale; R, 100–120 $\mu$m wide samples from outer half of stratum radiatum.

In animals L-7, cortex was removed also on the normal side (but without cutting the fimbria).

Lesions of the fimbria of rats have also been shown to produce a 32% decrease in whole brain ACh content after 3 days (Pepeu *et al.*, 1973).

In behavioural studies, it has been shown that both hippocampal lesions (e.g. Racine and Kimble, 1965) and intra-hippocampal injections of carbachol (Greene and Lomax, 1970) produce impairment of learning. Impairment of passive-avoidance learning in mice, produced either by bilateral hippocampal lesions or by intra-ventricular injections of ChAc inhibitors, was correlated with decreases in ChAc activity of the hippocampus (Glick *et al.*, 1973). In these studies, intra-peritoneal injections of scopolamine potentiated the behavioural effects of both treatments. Glick *et al.*, (1973) concluded that the release of newly-synthesized ACh at hippocampal synapses might be essential for passive avoidance learning. However, a functional role for the hippocampus in learning and memory remains unclear. For example, performance of a brightness discrimination task by cats, which was usually accompanied by hippocampal "theta" activity, was not affected by direct injections of scopolamine into the medial septal nucleus which caused a marked reduction in theta activity (Bennett, 1973). But, it does seem clear that cholinergic mechanisms are implicated in septo-hippocampal functions.

## C. Role of the Reticular Formation

The midline thalamic nuclei appear to be associated with non-specific motivational processes which seem to be governed by the animal's level of arousal. Gastaut (1958) has suggested that the thalamic and brain stem reticular formation may serve as an essential link in pathways responsible for learning, recall and retention. In this connection, Grossman *et al.* (1965) showed that cholinergic stimulation of midline and reticular nuclei of the thalamus interfered with recently-learned behaviour in appetitive and aversive situations. In further work, Grossman and Peters (1966) showed that implantation of crystalline N-methyl-atropine nitrate into rat thalamic reticular nuclei impaired performance during acquisition and at asymptote in appetitive (black-white maze discrimi-nation) and aversive (shuttle-box avoidance) situations which indicated that this area may be involved in associative or memory processes (Fig. 5.17). On the other hand, implantations of this agent into midline thalamic nuclei facilitated behaviour under both of the above situations. Since specific motivational processes or simple sensory-motor functions were not affected by the injections of N-methyl-atropine into lateral or midline thalamic nuclei, it was concluded that cholinergic mechanisms in the thalamus might be related to non-specific motivational processes. Lesions produced by implantation of cannulae into the mesencephalic reticular formation (MRF): (1) reduced performance of a simple avoidance response; (2) did not affect instrumental escape responses; (3) facilitated acquisition and performance of simple appetitive habits (Grossman, 1966b; Grossman and Grossman, 1966; see Figs 2.6 and 5.18). Initial or infrequently-repeated cholinergic stimulation of the MRF in these same rats caused more severe impairment of avoidance and appetitive responses, while opposite effects were caused by fre-quently-repeated stimulation.

TABLE 15. Rate (presses/min.) of lever pressing for food- or water-rewards during a 30 min. test period. Reproduced with permission from Grossman (1968).

| Substance and amount injected | Food | | Water | |
|---|---|---|---|---|
| | $D^1$ | $C^1$ | $D^1$ | $C^1$ |
| **Carbachol chloride** | | | | |
| 0·5 μg | 15·8[b] | 42·1 | 19·1[b] | 35·9 |
| 1·0 μg | 10·1[b] | 44·3 | 17·4[b] | 34·5 |
| 1·5 μg | 7·9[b] | 40·8 | 8·1[b] | 35·0 |
| 2·0 μg | 2·1[b] | 41·7 | 1·5[b] | 36·7 |
| 2·0 μg in solution | 4·9[b] | 45·1 | 0·0[b] | 34·8 |
| **Acetylcholine chloride** | | | | |
| 2·0 μg | 39·1 | 44·3 | 35·8 | 36·6 |
| 4·0 μg | 37·4 | 40·7 | 32·3 | 37·1 |
| 8·0 μg | 34·1[a] | 42·9 | 29·1[a] | 35·4 |
| 8·0 μg in solution | 38·1 | 46·3 | 29·7[a] | 36·8 |
| **Atropine sulfate** | | | | |
| 2·0 μg | 44·1 | 47·1 | 33·0 | 32·3 |
| 6·0 μg | 39·1 | 46·3 | 28·1 | 34·1 |
| 12·0 μg | 33·3[a] | 45·9 | 20·1[b] | 35·5 |
| 12·0 μg in solution | 36·0[a] | 46·7 | 24·0[b] | 36·0 |
| **Nor-adrenaline bitartrate** | | | | |
| 2·0 μg | 40·0 | 46·7 | 31·1 | 36·0 |
| 4·0 μg | 34·4[a] | 44·0 | 25·9[b] | 34·8 |
| 8·0 μg | 29·1[a] | 45·5 | 21·1[a] | 35·7 |
| 8·0 μg in solution | 31·3[a] | 46·1 | 20·1[a] | 34·9 |
| **Dibenzyline** | | | | |
| 2·0 μg | 42·8 | 41·7 | 37·1 | 38·1 |
| 8·0 μg | 47·7 | 43·3 | 44·8[a] | 37·6 |
| 16·0 μg | 47·2[a] | 42·9 | 45·1 | 39·2 |
| 16·0 μg in solution | 48·0[a] | 42·1 | 44·1 | 39·0 |

[a] $p < 0.005$.
[b] $p < 0.001$.

$D^1$, average of 2 drug tests; $C^1$, average of 2 control tests. Substances were injected directly into the MRF of rats. Note that carbachol implants or injections, which caused hyper-reactivity to sensory inputs, were most effective at lowering the rate of responding for both food and water rewards in the 2-lever operant conditioning apparatus. Nor-adrenaline, on the other hand, generally decreased the animals reactivity to environmental stimuli; this was also reflected as a depression of both food- and water-rewarded behaviour.

Grossman (1968) showed also that application of cholinergic agents directly to the MRF interfered with acquisition and with the execution of conditioned responses in various appetitive test situations, while not affecting relevant motivational processes (e.g. hunger, thirst) and sensory or motor functioning. It was suggested that cholinergic substances produced a pattern of behavioural changes which seemed to be due to a sharply increased level of reactivity to sensory input in all modalities, and that the interference with acquisition and execution of conditioned responses might have been due to the animal's inability to restrict its "attention" to relevant aspects of the environment (see Table 15). These ideas seem to be in accord with the hypothesis of Carlton (1963) that the central cholinergic system may be involved in the mediation of the effects of "non-reward". These studies, taken together with those in which it was shown that intra-amygdalar injections of scopolamine facilitated (Belluzzi and Grossman, 1969), and that carbachol or eserine injections inhibited (Belluzzi, 1972) one-way avoidance acquisition, indicate that cholinergic mechanisms in the reticular formation as well as in the amygdala-hippocampus and septal regions may be involved in the regulation of motivation and learning.

### D. *Other Studies on Avoidance Behaviours*

It has also been shown that the anti-avoidance actions of chlorpromazine and of some other major tranquilizers (e.g. perphenazine) can be reversed by systemic injections of various anti-cholinergic agents (e.g. benztropine) in squirrel monkeys (Hanson *et al.*, 1970; see also Jenny and Healy, 1959, and Fig. 5.19). These data have added support to earlier findings that ChE-inhibitors potentiated the anti-avoidance effects of perphenazine (Proctor *et al.*, 1964; Goldberg and Johnson, 1964), and that ChE inhibitors (Goldberg *et al.*, 1965) and arecoline (Chalmers and Erickson, 1964) possessed anti-avoidance activity. On the other hand, the anti-avoidance activities of agents having central sedative-hypnotic properties (e.g. chlordiazepoxide, pentobarbital and chloral hydrate) were increased by concurrent administration of benztropine in squirrel monkeys (Hanson *et al.*, 1970). These studies have provided further, but indirect, evidence for the involvement of central cholinergic agents in mechanisms of learning, and in the possible etiologies of emotional and mental disturbances of man.

### E. *Self-stimulation Behaviour*

Another operant behaviour which has received a great deal of attention with relation to its possible mediation by central cholinergic mechanisms is self-stimulation (see e.g. Olds and Milner, 1954; Brady, 1961; Olds, 1962). Self-stimulation involves the concept of "pleasure-eliciting centres" of the brain (see e.g. Olds, 1958); i.e. the animal learns to stimulate certain areas of its own brain to obtain electrical reinforcement ("reward"). This behaviour may be elicited from many areas of the brain in rats, monkeys and other animals, but the exact anatomy of intra-cranial self-stimulation has not been clarified in rats (see e.g. Wetzel, 1968), or in monkeys (see e.g. Routtenberg, 1971). Among the cerebral structures which have been involved in self-stimulation behaviour are, hypothalamic areas, medial forebrain bundle, septal areas, medial edge of the internal capsule, zona incerta and stria

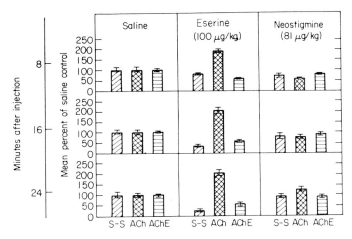

FIG. 5.21. A comparison of the effects of equimolar doses of eserine and neostigmine on self-stimulation behaviour, brain ACh content and AChE activity. The data were plotted for different groups of animals at 8, 16 and 24 min. after injection of saline, eserine or neostigmine. Note that eserine caused an increase in brain ACh, a decrease in brain AChE and a decrease in self-stimulation behaviour (*S-S*) while neostigmine had relatively little effect. Behavioural data represent cumulative scores over 8 min. periods, whereas brain assays were made at the time of sacrifice. Reproduced with permission from Domino and Olds (1968).

medullaris. These regions of the brain contain appreciable amounts of cholinergic elements (see Figs 2.16–2.18, 3.4, 3.5, 4.6, 4.7).

Domino and Olds (1968) compared the effects of subcutaneous injections of the two anti-ChE agents, eserine and neostigmine, on self-stimulation in rats and correlated this behaviour with cerebral AChE activity and ACh content. It was shown that eserine (100 $\mu$g/kg, s.c.) produced a marked depressant effect on self-stimulation which was roughly correlated in time course with decreased cerebral AChE activity and increased cerebral ACh levels (Fig. 5.20). Since neostigmine, even in larger doses, did not alter appreciably cerebral ACh or AChE, it was suggested that this agent exerted mainly peripheral actions (see also Stark and Boyd, 1963; Fig. 5.21). It was concluded that central cholinergic systems were involved in inhibiting electrical self-stimulation of the lateral hypothalamus. It should be noted that increases in brain ACh caused by AChE inhibitors have also been correlated with changes

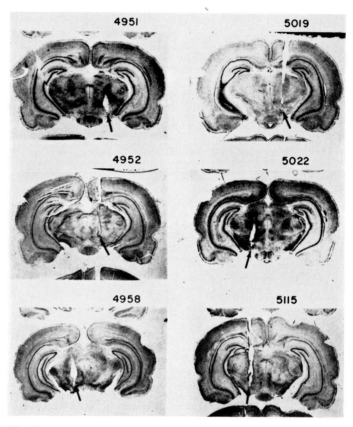

Fig. 5.22. Histologic sections of posterior lateral hypothalamic "rewarding" regions of rat brain. Frozen sections were cut transversely 50 $\mu$ thick and stained with cresyl violet. Regions below the tips of electrode tracks (*arrows*) are where electric shock produced positive reinforcing behaviour. Reproduced with permission from Olds and Domino (1969a).

in the EEG and in ACh release from the cerebral cortex (e.g. see §2.2 and Chapter 6). The behavioural inhibition caused in these studies could have been related to an increased interaction of ACh with its receptors, or to an altered sensitivity of hypothalamic neurones caused by ACh accumulation in the brain. Further studies by Olds and Domino (1969a) led them to conclude that muscarinic cholinergic agonists which penetrate the "blood-brain barrier" depress posterior lateral hypothalamic self-stimulation on a central basis, while nicotinic cholinergic agonists have complex depressant and stimulant effects, both centrally and peripherally (see Fig. 5.22). It was shown also that escape behaviour (elicited by electrical stimulation of the midbrain tegmentum) was not inhibited by subcutaneous administration of cholinergic agonists (e.g. eserine, arecoline) in doses which inhibited hypothalamic self-stimulation ("approach") behaviour (Olds and Domino, 1969b; Fig. 5.23).

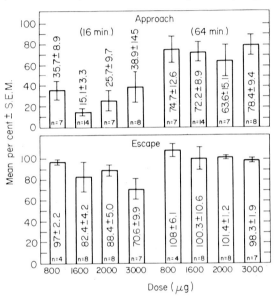

Fig. 5.23. Dose-effect relationships between arecoline and approach (self-stimulation) or escape behaviour for electrical stimulation of the brain in rats. The effects of arecoline (800–3000 $\mu$g/kg, s.c.) on approach behaviour induced by electrical stimulation of the lateral posterior hypothalamus were compared with those on escape behaviour elicited by electrical stimulation of the midbrain tegmentum. Note that larger doses of arecoline were required to depress escape behaviour than were needed to depress approach behaviour. Means $\pm$ S.E.M. of percentage change from control after various doses of arecoline, at the time of peak drug effect (16 min.), and during recovery (64 min., post-injection); four or more rats per group. Reproduced with permission from Olds and Domino (1969b).

In more recent studies with rats trained to self-stimulate for electrical "reward" in the posterior lateral hypothalamus, it was shown that *d*-amphetamine facilitated low rates of self-stimulation, while inhibiting high rates (Domino and Olds, 1972). In these experiments administration of amphetamine tended to cause decreases in cerebral ACh content. Scopolamine has also been shown to have a rate-dependent effect on behaviour (Domino and Olds, 1972; see also McKim, 1973; Houser and Houser, 1973).

*F. Possible Cholinergic Roles in Learning and Memory*

The perseveration-consolidation theory of learning and memory, i.e. that "neural traces" which represent elements "to-be-associated" might perseverate as a closed "reverberatory" system for a period of time after cessation of stimulation and then may become consolidated to form memory (see Hilgard and Marquis, 1940; Konorski, 1948; Hebb, 1949; Gerard, 1949; Gomulicki, 1953; John, 1967), has received much support from results obtained in studies of the effects of pre- and post-trial injections of convulsant and anti-ChE agents on learning (see e.g. McGaugh and Petrinovich, 1959, 1965; Breen and McGaugh, 1961; McGaugh and Thomson, 1962; Petrinovich, 1963; McGaugh, 1968). This "memory trace" or "consolidation" type of theory has stemmed from the early work of Lorente de Nó (1938) and has received further support from neurophysiological studies which indicated that reverberatory activity might exist in isolated slabs of cerebral cortex (Burns, 1954, 1958). Also, "trace" theory appears to be the most successful way to explain the retrograde amnesia (disturbance of retention) which occurs when animals are subjected to electro-convulsive shock, cerebral concussion or anoxia during, or shortly after, learning (Duncan, 1949; Glickman, 1961; McGaugh, 1966). In this connection, it seems interesting that ACh has been found in the CSF only in humans subjected to craniocerebral trauma or electro-convulsive shock or in some epileptics (Tower and MacEachern, 1949a, b).

With regard to the cholinergic system, it has been shown that acquisition rates in animals are increased by treatment with anti-ChE agents (Platt, 1951; Russell, 1954) and that post-trial injections of eserine facilitate the rate of maze learning in rats (Stratton and Petrinovich, 1963). These findings led Stratton and Petrinovich (1963) to suggest that the ratio of ACh/ChE in the brain was an index of the probable time course of perseverative neural activity. However, the effects of anti-ChE agents differ with regard to the time of their pre- or post-trial administration to rodents (e.g. Bureš *et al.*, 1962; Jennings, 1963; Doty and Johnston, 1966; Deutsch and Leibowitz, 1966; Whitehouse, 1966; Wiener and Deutsch, 1968; Squire, 1970; Squire *et al.*, 1971; Warburton and Brown, 1972; Izquierdo *et al.*, 1973), and in certain learning tasks both central and peripheral actions of eserine appear to affect performance in mice (Squire *et al.*, 1971). Glassman (1969) has recently reviewed the literature about the relationship between cerebral ACh and the possible amnesic effects of diisopropyl-fluorophosphate (DFP) and eserine (see also Deutsch *et al.*, 1966; Hamburg, 1967) and has mentioned the findings that anti-cholinergic agents, like atropine or scopolamine, also affect recall. The temporal variations in amnesia produced by DFP have been interpreted in terms of the synaptic action of ACh (see Deutsch and Rocklin, 1967).

In rats it has also been shown that scopolamine can produce amnesia (Pazzagli and Pepeu, 1964). Both DFP and scopolamine produce amnesia, but by different mechanisms. Scopolamine has been shown to produce its greatest amnesias for habits of the ages at which the effects of DFP were least marked and *vice versa* (Deutscq and Rocklin, 1967). In a recent article, Deutsch (1971) has hypothesized, on the basis of drug studies, that post-synaptic endings at a specific set of synapses become more sensitive to transmitter as a result of learning and that this sensitivity increases with time after initial learning and then declines. He stated further that synaptic conductance is altered by learning and that cholinergic synapses are modified by learning (i.e. that post-synaptic membranes become increasingly more sensitive to ACh with time after learning) and that both original learning and extinction are subserved by cholinergic synapses. Perhaps his most interesting finding was that either facilitation, or impairment, of memory could be produced in rats (subjected to simple learning tasks) with the same dose of anti-ChE simply as a function of time of injection after original learning, as might be expected if changes in the biochemical structure of synapses formed the substrate of memory (see also §5.4). Perhaps the major problems which exist for consolidation theory are: (1) the highly variable results obtained for amnesia gradients with post-trial electro-convulsive shock (e.g. Heriot and Coleman, 1962; Chorova and Schiller, 1965; McGaugh, 1966); and (2) whether or not short- and long-term memory traces do indeed exist (see Wickelgren, 1973). Mah and Albert (1973) have suggested that differences in task characteristics and in electroshock parameters appear to account for most of the variation found in estimating amnesia gradients.

### 5.4 Environmental Effects on Central Cholinergic Mechanisms

It is now well known that changes in environment, as well as changes in maturation and nutrition, affect cerebral physiological and biochemical mechanisms which are involved in the central control behaviour (see e.g. Roberts and Matthysse, 1970, and Fig. 5.24). For excellent reviews of the early theories which have related changes in experience to changes in cerebral structure, chemistry and physiology, see Bennett *et al.*, (1964) and Kandel and Spencer (1968). Since the respiratory quotient (R.Q.) of the brains of man and most experimental mammals is about 1·0 (see e.g. Elliott and Wolfe, 1962; Bradford, 1968; Quastel, 1969; Balazs, 1970), and since a decreased utilization of glucose (i.e. decreased glucose tolerance) was perhaps the first biochemical symptom of "mental depression" ever measured in humans (Kooy, 1919; Mann,

1925), it seems obvious that carbohydrate metabolism is involved in many, if not all, of the behavioural changes which occur in man (see references in Shopsin *et al.*, 1972). These were significant findings in that cerebral glucose is also the major precursor for the acetyl groups necessary for ACh synthesis in the brain. It has been shown that labelled ACh appears rapidly in the brain after systemic injections of labelled precursors of acetyl-CoA (e.g. Cheney *et al.*, 1969; Tuček and Cheng, 1970) and that ACh is readily formed from glucose and pyruvate in brain slices (e.g. Browning and Schulman, 1968; Nakamura *et al.*, 1970; Lefresne *et al.*, 1973). Also glucose carbon-atom incorporation into the

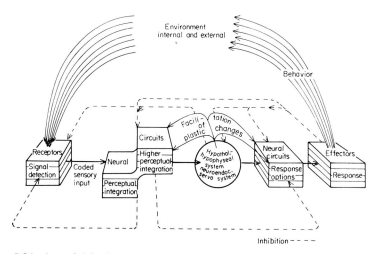

Fig. 5.24. A model for behaviour showing the major systems involved in informational transactions. Note that experience of the external and internal environments by the organism occurs only through sensory receptors and that the processing of this information by the nervous system results in reactions of the organism to, and/or upon, the environment which make up the emitted behaviour. Reproduced with permission from Roberts and Matthysse (1970).

brain was decreased markedly in mice which had been subjected to isolation-rearing (e.g. DeFeudis, 1971, 1972, 1973, 1974). Such "isolation" of mice also causes marked changes in their behaviour (e.g. Allee, 1942; Ginsberg and Allee, 1942; Welch, 1965). These findings indicate, on an indirect basis, that ACh synthesis from glucose should be altered by environmental changes which affect the animal's level of experience and hence, its behaviour.

With more specific regard to the central cholinergic system, it has been shown that subjecting rats to environmental enrichment, during development produced changes in brain AChE and ChE activities which were paralleled by improvement on learning tasks (e.g. Krech *et al.*, 1960, 1962a, b, 1963, 1966; Bennett *et al.*, 1964; Rosenzweig *et al.*, 1967; Bennett and Rosenzweig, 1971; see Fig. 5.25). On the basis of these studies it was postulated that these changes in central cholinergic activity might be involved in learning. Also, electro-shock treatment of rats during development impairs learning and also alters central ChE and AChE activities (e.g. Pryor *et al.*, 1966, 1967). An investigation by Brown (1971) of the pattern and duration of changes in brain ChE and

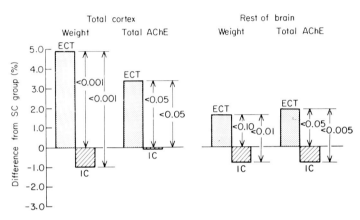

Fig. 5.25. Comparisons among values for brain weight and total AChE activity of littermate rats maintained under *ECT* (environmental complexity and training), *SC* (standard colony) or *IC* (isolated) conditions from 105–185 days of age. Differences from *SC* values are expressed as percentages of *SC* values; $p$-values indicate significant differences. Both the total weight and the total AChE activity of the cerebral cortex were increased by subjecting the rats to *ECT*, but since the relative increase in AChE was less than that for tissue weight the *ECT* values were lower than *IC* values when AChE was expressed per unit tissue weight. Reproduced with permission from Bennett *et al.*, (1964).

AChE produced by long- and short-term exposure of rats to enriched environments has indicated that the changes in these enzymes that follow both short- and long-term treatments which give rise to learning do not persist as long as the observed behavioural changes. This finding is inconsistent with the postulated cholinergic involvement, in a purely quantitative manner, in long-term memory storage and retrieval. Other studies have indicated that a correlation exists between brain AChE levels and functional state and adaptive behaviour (Rogers *et al.*, 1960; Burdick and Strittmatter, 1965; Saunders, 1966; Vernadakis and Burkhalter, 1967). However, Consolo and Valzelli (1970) have not been able to show changes in ChAc activity in whole brain or brain regions of mice made aggressive by 30 days of environmental isolation.

Another line of evidence which indicates that cholinergic mechanisms may be involved in functional roles of the nervous system stems from the recent work concerning hormonal influences on brain ChE (AChE + pseudo-ChE) activity. McKinney (1970) studied brain ChE levels in "grouped" versus "singly-caged" adrenal-demedullated rats, and showed that adrenal-demedullation produced a decrease in the brain AChE activity of singly-caged animals. With group-housed animals, brain AChE activity was increased in adrenal-demedullated, but not altered in intact animals. Total brain ChE activity was correlated with the brain weight of intact, but not of adrenal-demedullated, animals. This worker suggested that hormones of the adrenal medulla may be involved in the stabilization of brain ChE activity during different environmental conditions. This work reflects back on earlier work concerning the effects of primary learning (environmental complexity) on brain AChE activity and brain weight (see above). Increases in group size also causes heavier adrenal glands (Christian, 1963) and increased catecholamine content of the adrenal medulla (Welch, 1965, 1967; Welch and Welch, 1968). In a review by Welch (1965) it was suggested that peripheral catecholamines might be involved in regulating the tonic activity of the reticular formation.

Karczmar (1969) has evaluated critically the studies which have shown the relationship between central cholinergic systems and behaviour. He has stressed the fact that in the studies of Krech *et al.*, (1962a, b, 1966) and Rosenzweig *et al.*, (1967) the differences in cerebral AChE caused by environmental alterations were only of the order of a few per cent (see Fig. 5.25) and that when expressed on a unit weight basis (see Bennett *et al.*, 1964) brain AChE activity was decreased by environmental enrichment. However, this should not be taken to mean that changes in cholinergic synapses were not caused by environmental changes. Bennett *et al.*, (1964), themselves, suggested that the decrease in AChE activity per unit weight of cerebral cortex might indicate that growth of the cortex caused by experience (environmental stimulation) could occur mainly in elements which are low in AChE activity (e.g. glia, non-cholinergic neurones). It seems necessary to carry out further studies in order to demonstrate, in a more conclusive fashion, these cerebral changes which can be produced by changing the level of experience of experimental animals. Further studies along this line should be encouraged.

Recently, it has been shown that environmental manipulations can modify the fine structure of cerebral neurones and glia (e.g. Diamond *et al.*, 1964, 1966; Globus and Scheibel, 1967; Altman, 1967; Valverde, 1967; Walsh *et al.*, 1969; Volkmar and Greenough, 1972; Globus *et al.*, 1972). Explanations for these environmental effects on cerebral morphology have included changes in dendritic branching, number of dendritic spines, total number of dendrites-plus-axonal arborizations. From these suggestions, Chronister *et al.*, (1973) concluded that the number of synaptic boutons should be the most sensitive measure of changes in axo-dendritic relationships. In their studies, it was shown that an increase in synaptic boutons occurred in the rat hippocampus during ontogenetic and environmental changes. This study has provided evidence that age and/or experience can alter the synaptic morphology of the hippocampus, a finding which is in line with the "neurophysiological postulate" of Hebb (1949) in which he stated:

> The most obvious and I believe much the most probable suggestion concerning the way in which one cell could become more capable of firing another is that synaptic knobs develop and increase the area of contact between the afferent axon and efferent soma.

In support of the notion that these morphological changes may be correlated with the cholinergic system, Essman (1971) has shown that individual housing ("isolation") of male mice for 165 days caused significant decreases in the "bound"/"free" ratio of ACh in their cerebral cortices which were paralleled by deficits in their acquisition of both passive and active conditioned avoidance responses (see Table 9). Also, prior treatment of mice with nicotine improved acquisition in isolated mice while impairing that of group-housed mice; in isolated mice nicotine increased the "bound"/"free" ratio of ACh in the cortex (Table 9). In further studies (Essman, 1972) it was shown that isolation of mice caused significant elevations in the ACh content of cerebral cortical homogenates and nerve-ending particles. These findings may be useful in relating central cholinergic systems to changes in arousal level which are known to occur in "isolated" animals (see Welch, 1965).

In sum, since changes in behaviour have been correlated with changes in cerebral glucose metabolism and with changes in cerebral cholinergic systems, and since the changes in behaviour can be produced by environmental manipulations which appear to alter cerebral synaptic morphology, it seems that such a combined approach may well lead to an explanation of the roles which the central cholinergic system may play in the regulation of behaviour. It seems interesting that D. O. Hebb had stressed the importance of such an approach about 25 years ago: "Our problem, then, is to find valid 'molar' conceptions of neural action (conceptions, i.e. that can be applied to large-scale cortical organizations)."

*Chapter 6*

# Supporting Studies on The Central Release of Acetylcholine

## 6.1 Introduction

Although a basic criterion which is thought to be necessary for conclusive identification of a neurotransmitter substance is the demonstration of its "release" from pre-synaptic terminals (see e.g. Eccles, 1964; Werman, 1966, 1972; Phillis, 1970), this has never been accomplished at a central synapse. In this chapter, the central release of ACh and the release mechanism, itself, will be discussed. Experimental data, obtained in various laboratories, will be evaluated in an attempt to provide some insight into whether ACh is a central transmitter and whether its release from central neurones can be studied effectively with presently-available methods. The writer would like to emphasize the idea that "collectability" of a substance does not necessarily imply that it has been "physiologically released". However, studies on the central release of ACh have provided much insight into mechanisms which are involved in the regulation of CNS function and behaviour, and therefore these will be presented in some detail.

The initial experiments on the central release of ACh were conducted by Elliott *et al.*, (1950) and by MacIntosh and Oborin (1953). Results obtained in these studies and in more recent ones (see e.g. Mitchell, 1963; Szerb, 1964, 1967; Delgado and Rubinstein, 1964; Phillis and Chong, 1965; Celesia and Jasper, 1966; Collier and Mitchell, 1966, 1967; Bartolini and Pepeu, 1967; Phillis, 1968a; Bartolini *et al.*, 1972) have supported the idea that some types of central excitation and inhibition may be mediated by cholinergic mechanisms. By using perfusion fluids containing anti-ChE agents, ACh has been collected from many structures of the CNS (see reviews by Hebb and Krnjević, 1962; 1962; Mitchell, 1966; Pepeu, 1972). However, in no study which has been conducted to date has it been possible to exclude extra-synaptic origins of the ACh collected. The ubiquitous nature of glial cells, along with the tissue damage, changes in blood or CSF pressure and changes in the level of anaesthesia which may occur during experiments, are among the many factors which can affect the collectability of ACh.

## 6.2 *In vivo* Studies

### A. Cerebral Cortex

Many studies have been conducted in efforts to learn more about the nature of ACh release from the cerebral cortex and about the possible involvements of centrally active agents with these mechanisms. It has been shown that atropine and scopolamine (e.g. Mitchell, 1963; Szerb, 1964; Celesia and Jasper, 1966; Bartolini and Pepeu, 1967; Beani *et al.*, 1968; Dudar and Szerb, 1969; Bartolini *et al.*, 1972; Aquilonius *et al.*, 1972), angiotensin (Elie and Panisset, 1970), pentylenetetrazol (e.g. Mitchell, 1963; Beleslin *et al.*, 1965; Celesia and Jasper, 1966; Hemsworth and Neal, 1968), nicotine (Armitage *et al.*, 1969), amphetamines (Pepeu and Bartolini, 1968; Deffenu *et al.*, 1970; Bartolini and Pepeu, 1970; Nistri *et al.*, 1972), picrotoxin (Szerb *et al.*, 1970) and both isomers of the psychotomimetic agent, Ditran (Domino and Bartolini, 1972) cause increases in ACh release from the cortex. On the other hand, narcotic analgesics, such as morphine (Beleslin and Polak, 1965; Beani *et al.*, 1968; Jhamandas *et al.*, 1970, 1971), the ganglionic blocking agent, hexamethonium-3 (Rao *et al.*, 1970; Szerb *et al.*, 1970), and other CNS depressants such as pentobarbital (MacIntosh and Oborin, 1953; Mitchell, 1963; Collier and Mitchell, 1967; Pepeu and Bartolini, 1968; Beani *et al.*, 1968), ethyl alcohol (Graham and Erickson, 1971), $\Delta^9$-THC (Domino and Bartolini, 1972) and chloralose (MacIntosh and Oborin, 1953; Mitchell, 1963) cause reductions in cortical ACh release. In addition, pronounced increases in cortical ACh release have been produced by traumatic brain injury in dogs (Metz, 1971b).

Mitchell (1963) and Szerb (1964) showed that ACh release from the mammalian cerebral cortex can be increased by systemically-administered or topically-applied atropine. This finding, taken with the evidence of Krnjević and Phillis (1963b) that atropine inhibits ACh-induced firing in cortical cholinoceptive cells, indicated that ACh release might be controlled by muscarinic receptors (see review by Mitchell, 1966). In a classic study, Celesia and Jasper (1966) examined both the EEG and the ACh release from the cortical surface of the un-anaesthetized (curarized) "dozing" cat during the application of various drugs or during electrical stimulation of the reticular formation. It was found that upon irrigation of the cortical surface with a solution containing neostigmine, the EEG was changed from the "sleep" pattern to a pattern of activity similar to that which is seen during "arousal".

However, neither the arousal-like EEG nor the epileptiform discharges which followed, altered the rate of ACh release so long as a stable state of sleep was maintained (Fig. 6.1). These results indicated that the desynchronization of the EEG caused by neostigmine differed from that caused by electrical stimulation of the mesencephalic reticular formation (e.g. Kanai and Szerb, 1965; Szerb, 1967) or by intravenous injection of metrazol (e.g. Mitchell, 1963), since in the latter two cases ACh release was increased. Celesia and Jasper (1966) suggested that neostigmine might act by stimulating intra-cortical cholinoceptive neurones, whereas stimulation of the reticular formation and metrazol injection might

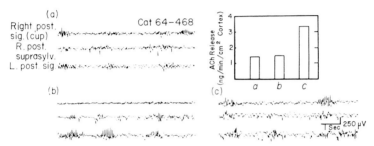

FIG. 6.1. Correlation of electrical activity and ACh release from the cerebral cortex. (*a*) Animal in normal drowsy state, during which sleep spindles are present over all cortical areas; (*b*) 60 min. later, the cortical area perfused with neostigmine shows fast asynchronous activity while ACh output is unchanged; (*c*) about 4 min. after administration of atropine (1 mg/kg, i.v.), cortical activation is blocked, slow waves and sleep spindles reappear over the perfused area, and ACh output is considerably increased. Reproduced with permission from Celesia and Jasper (1966).

activate afferent cholinergic fibres to these neurones. Perhaps the most striking observation made during this study was that atropine (1 mg/kg, i.v.) strongly enhanced ACh release from both resting and stimulated cortex while producing a "sleeplike" EEG pattern (Figs 6.1 and 6.2; see also Kanai and Szerb, 1965).

In agreement with the results of Celesia and Jasper (1966), Bartolini and Pepeu (1967) showed, in cats transected at either the midpontine, pre-trigeminal level ("desynchronized" EEG) or at the collicular level ("synchronized" EEG), that a greater amount of ACh was released from the cortex during desynchronization of the EEG (Fig. 6.3; see also Table 1). Administration of hyoscine, either intravenously (Fig. 6.4) or by its addition to collection fluids (Fig. 6.5), greatly increased ACh output. Application of local anaesthetic agents decreased both the spontaneous release of ACh and the effects of hyoscine. These findings support further the notion that atropine-like substances may cause

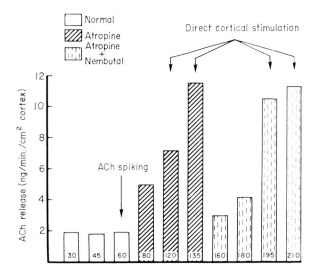

Fig. 6.2. Release of ACh from the primary somato-sensory cortex of the cat. The first two columns represent the ACh ouput in the normal waking animal; other columns represent the effects of ACh spiking, atropine, Nembutal, and direct cortical stimulation on the amount of ACh released. The numbers on the abscissa represent the time (min.) after the beginning of cortical perfusion with physiological solution containing neostigmine. Reproduced with permission from Celesia and Jasper (1966).

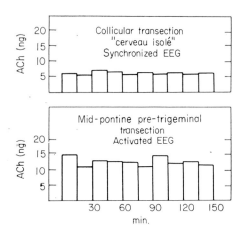

Fig. 6.3. The output of ACh (expressed as ng/15 min./cm²) from the cat somato-sensory cortex. Cats were transected at the collicular or mid-pontine, pre-trigeminal level; 15 min. collection periods. Reproduced with permission from Bartolini and Pepeu (1967).

increases in ACh release by their interaction with central muscarinic receptors (see also Giarman and Pepeu, 1964; Deffenu *et al.*, 1966).

Dudar and Szerb (1969) studied further the effects of local application of atropine on the resting and evoked release of ACh from cat cerebral

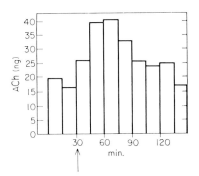

FIG. 6.4. Effect of intravenous administration of 0·75 mg/kg hyoscine HBr (*arrow*) on ACh output (expressed as ng/15 min./cm*I*) from the parietal cortex of a cat transected at the mid-pontine, pre-trigeminal level. Reproduced with permission from Bartolini and Pepeu (1967).

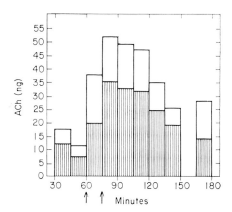

FIG. 6.5. Effect of 1 μg hyoscine HBr, added to collecting cups, on the output of ACh from the somato-sensory cortex of the right (*white*) and left (*shaded*) hemispheres of a cat transected at the mid-pontine, pre-trigeminal level and hemisected on the left side at the collicular level. Hyoscine was added during the time indicated by the arrows; ACh output is expressed as ng/15 min./cm². Reproduced with permission from Bartolini and Pepeu (1967).

cortex using "Dial" (allobarbitone + urethane) or halothane-$N_2O$ anaesthesia. ACh release occurred to a greater extent with "Dial" than with the gaseous anaesthetic (cf. Phillis, 1968a; see below); addition of atropine (1 μg/ml) to the fluid within the perfusion cup increased ACh release by about 4-fold in cats anaesthetized with "Dial" but had no effect on those anaesthetized with halothane-$N_2O$ (Fig. 6.6). Cortical undercutting, mesencephalic lesions or topically-applied tetrodotoxin (TTX) reduced or abolished both resting and atropine-induced ACh release (see also Szerb, 1967; Bartolini and Pepeu, 1967; Bjegović *et al.*, 1969). ACh release by electrical stimulation of the reticular formation of cats under halothane-$N_2O$ anaesthesia was increased about 4-fold by

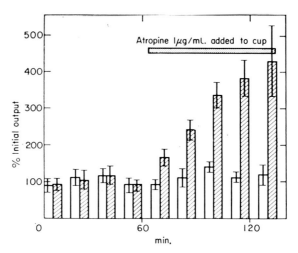

FIG. 6.6. Average resting ACh output under "Dial" hatched bars or halothane-$N_2O$ open bars anaesthesia, and the effect of topically-applied atropine. To normalize results, in each experiment values for ACh output before atropine were pooled and individual outputs were expressed as percentages of these pooled values. (This applies also to Fig. 6.7.) Averages $\pm$ S.E.M. of percentages are indicated. The overall average values before atropine were: halothane-$N_2O$, $100\% = 0.26$ ng/cm²/min. (n = 3); "Dial", $100\% = 2.23$ ng/cm²/min. (n = 8). Reproduced with permission from Dudar and Szerb (1969).

atropine, but with direct cortical stimulation it was increased only about 2-fold. Atropine had no effect on the release of ACh which was produced by topical application of KCl (cf. Polak's (1971) results with brain slices; see below). Interestingly, atropine also caused an increase in the output of ACh from the contralateral cortex, but this was not as pronounced as that from the ipsilateral cortex (Fig. 6.7). It seems possible that the greater ACh release caused by atropine from the ipsilateral cortex may have been due to its effects on both cortical electrical activity and muscarinic receptors, while the release from the contralateral side may have been due solely to changes in cortical electrical activity. Dudar and Szerb concluded that atropine caused increases in ACh release by

blocking cholinergic synapses which are involved in a negative feedback circuit controlling the activity of cholinergic neurones (see also
MacIntosh, 1963).

Stimulation of the mesencephalic reticular formation (MRF) has
been shown to enhance ACh release from all areas of the cortex which
have been tested (Kanai and Szerb, 1965; Celesia and Jasper, 1966;
Szerb, 1967; Phillis, 1968a). This lack of specificity of ACh release upon

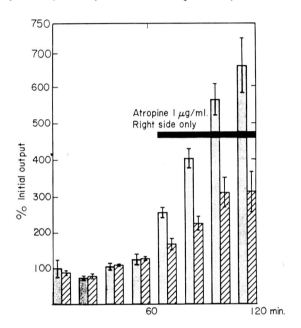

Fig. 6.7. Effect of direct unilateral application of atropine on average ipsilateral
and contralateral ACh outputs in "Dial"-anaesthetized cats. Grey bars, right side
(with atropine), 100% = 1·28 ng/cm²/min. (n = 3); ▨, left side (without atropine),
100% = 1·18 ng/cm²/min. (n = 3); horizontal black bar indicates application of
atropine. Reproduced with permission from Dudar and Szerb (1969).

reticular stimulation indicates that ACh is involved with the diverse
mechanisms and anatomical pathways underlying cortical arousal, and
correlates well with the results of histochemical studies on the distribution
of AChE (e.g. Lewis and Shute, 1967; Shute and Lewis, 1967). The
finding that reticular stimulation caused both EEG activation and
increased ACh release led Szerb (1967) to study the relationship between
these two phenomena. In Szerb's experiments, performed on halothane
-N₂O anaesthetized cats, the increase in cortical ACh release produced
by reticular stimulation was found to be greatest at frequencies of 30,
60 and 100/s, and stimulation at 60 and 100/s exerted maximal effects

on reducing low-frequency and on increasing high-frequency EEG
activities (Fig. 6.8). Acute cortical isolation reduced markedly the
evoked ACh release while not affecting resting release (Fig. 6.9). By
stimulating various sub-cortical areas (i.e. reticular formation, hypothalamus, medial thalamus, septum, dorsal hippocampus, caudate
nucleus) it was shown that cortical EEG activation and ACh release did

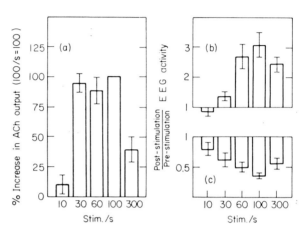

Fig. 6.8. (a) Increase in ACh release from the cerebral cortex during stimulation
of the reticular formation at different frequencies. Summary of experiments on eight
cats anaesthetized with halothane-$N_2O$. Each observation consists of the difference
between the output during stimulation and the resting output immediately preceding
it. In each experiment the increase at 100/s stimulation was compared with the effect
of 1–3 other frequencies and the increase due to 100/s stimulation was made equal to
100%. Each result is an average of 4 or 5 observations; S.E.M. indicated by vertical
lines. (b) Changes in high frequency EEG activity due to stimulation of the reticular
formation at different frequencies. Each bar represents an average of 5 observations
on one cat anaesthetized with halothane-$N_2O$. A train of 100 stimuli was delivered
every 4–5 min. at indicated frequencies, the order of frequencies being selected at
random. The vertical axis shows the ratio of activity 10 s following stimulation over
the activity 10 s immediately before stimulation; S.E.M. as above. (c) Changes in low
frequency EEG activity due to stimulation of the reticular formation. Results were
obtained simultaneously with those shown in (b); symbols as in (b). Reproduced with
permission from Szerb (1967).

not vary in a parallel fashion, and hence it was suggested that different
anatomical pathways are involved in these two phenomena (see Fig.
6.10). Further support for this apparent dissociation between EEG
activation and ACh release was derived from experiments on the action
of atropine (see above and Chapter 2). However, it seems evident that
both EEG activation and increased ACh release involve pathways which

reach the cortex by way of the mesencephalic tegmentum (see also Kanai and Szerb, 1965; Sie *et al.*, 1965; Celesia and Jasper, 1966).

Other experiments have indicated that the release of ACh from specific sensory receiving areas of the cerebral cortex can be enhanced by stimulating appropriate sensory pathways (Mitchell, 1963; Collier and Mitchell, 1966, 1967; Hemsworth and Mitchell, 1969). Collier and Mitchell (1966) found, in Dial-anaesthetized rabbits, that photic

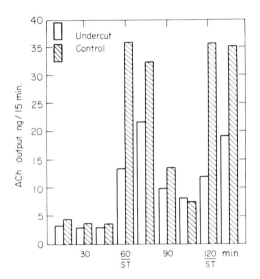

FIG. 6.9. Release of ACh from normal and undercut cortices during electrical stimulation of the reticular formation (cat under halothane-N₂O anaesthesia). *Unfilled bars*, ACh output from undercut (*left*) cortex; *hatched bars*, ACh output from normal (*right*) cortex. Periods of electrical stimulation are indicated. Reproduced with permission from Szerb (1967).

stimulation of the retina or electrical stimulation of the ipsilateral lateral geniculate body (LGB) caused a greater increase in ACh release from primary visual cortex than from other areas of the cortex (Fig. 6.11). Electrical stimulation of the visual pathway also produced an increase in ACh release from the contralateral visual cortex but this was slight compared to that on the ipsilateral side (Fig. 6.12). Since the evoked release of ACh from the contralateral cortex was not abolished by sectioning the transcallosal pathway, it was suggested that this response was mediated by another pathway, i.e. perhaps by the ascending reticular pathway concerned with arousal. However, since cholinergic fibres originating in the reticular formation may pass through the LGB (see Deffenu *et al.*, 1967), the arousal pathway could have been involved in both the ipsi- and contra-lateral release of ACh. Also, it seems well established that stimulation of the MRF alters synaptic transmission through the LGB (see Doty *et al.*, 1973; Wilson *et al.*, 1973; Bartlett *et al.*, 1973). Collier and Mitchell (1966) concluded that two ascending

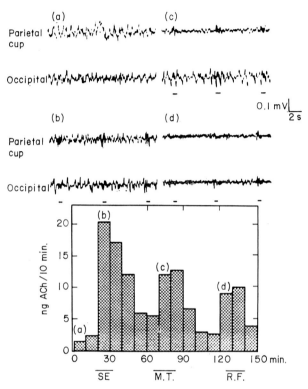

FIG. 6.10. EEG and cortical ACh release during stimulation of various subcortical sites in a cat anaesthetized with halothane-N$_2$O. Horizontal bars below records indicate stimulation at 100/s every 10 s throughout a 10 min. collection period. Letters above EEG tracings refer to the collection periods during which EEG tracings were obtained. Samples were collected and the EEG was recorded ipsilateral to stimulation. *SE*, septum; *M.T.*, medial thalamus; *R.F.*, reticular formation. Reproduced with permission from Szerb (1967).

cholinergic systems could account for these observations: (1) non-specific reticulo-cortical system, for widespread ACh release; (2) specific thalamo-cortical system, for ACh release from primary receiving areas of the cortex.

Further experiments on the effects of brain lesions on the release of ACh from the cerebral cortices of awake rabbits have supported the

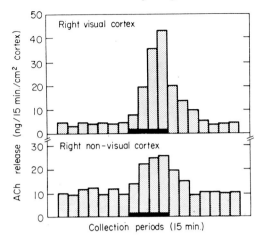

FIG. 6.11. Release of ACh from visual and non-visual areas of the cerebral cortex of a rabbit anaesthetized with "Dial" during photic stimulation of both eyes. Collecting cups were placed onto right visual receiving area and right non-visual area of the cortex. Periods of continuous photic stimulation are indicated by horizontal bars. Reproduced with permission from Collier and Mitchell (1966).

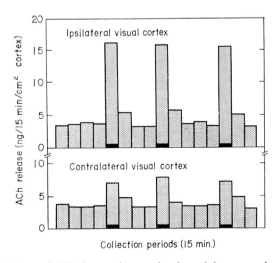

FIG. 6.12. Release of ACh from primary visual receiving areas during direct electrical stimulation of the left lateral geniculate body (rabbit anaesthetized with "Dial"). Collecting cups were placed onto left (*ipsilateral*) and right (*contralateral*) visual areas of the cortex. Periods of stimulation of the lateral geniculate body at 20/s are indicated by horizontal bars. Reproduced with permission from Collier and Mitchell (1966).

existence of two major ascending cholinergic systems (Collier and Mitchell, 1967; Fig. 6.13). These workers showed also that both the spontaneous and the evoked release of ACh (by direct electrical stimulation)
were reduced by chronic undercutting of the visual cortex and they
interpreted this as evidence for the presence of only a few, if any, cholinergic intra-corticaln eurones. This interpretation does not appear to be
entirely valid (see e.g. Phillis, 1968a). It seems more likely that the
decrease in spontaneous release of ACh from cortex which had been
undercut for 22 days was due to tissue degeneration and associated

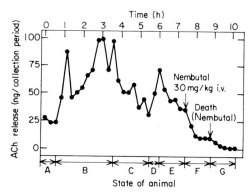

Fig. 6.13. Release of ACh from the visual cortex of a free-moving rabbit during
anaesthesia and consciousness (perfusion system implanted in left visual cortex).
Perfusion rate, 0·5 ml/15–18 min.; samples assayed on recovery of 0·5 ml of perfusate.
Allowance was made for dead space volume of collecting tube of 0·5 ml. Legend on
lower abscissa indicates the state of the animal as follows: (A) anaesthetized after
cannula implantation; (B) recovered from anaesthesia and continuously active,
exploring cage, eating and drinking; (C) quiet and moving only occasionally; (D)
active; (E) quiet; (F) anaesthetized after Nembutal (30 mg/kg, i.v.) at *arrow*; (G)
dead after lethal dose of Nembutal at *arrow*. Reproduced with permission from
Collier and Mitchell (1967).

metabolic changes and that spontaneously-released ACh, at least in
part, does not require sub-cortical afferent input (see e.g. Szerb, 1967
and Fig. 6.9). Evoked ACh release, on the other hand, does indeed seem
to depend on sub-cortical input (Collier and Mitchell, 1967; Szerb,
1967). However, this interpretation is complicated further by the use of
different anaesthetic agents; Collier and Mitchell (1967) used Dial and
Szerb (1967) used halothane-$N_2O$. In later work, Dudar and Szerb
(1969) showed, in Dial-anaesthetized cats, that even acute undercutting
can produce a substantial reduction of spontaneous ACh release. Hence,
spontaneously-released ACh may consist of two components, one within
the cortex, itself, which may be related to activation of local intra-
cortical circuits (e.g. Phillis and York, 1968; Jordan and Phillis, 1972),

and the other due to afferent subcortical input to the cortex. With Dial, both components may be active, but with halothane-$N_2O$ the subcortical component may be depressed (i.e. at the doses of these anaesthetics which were used in the experiments mentioned above). Hemsworth and Mitchell (1969) studied the characteristics of ACh release in the auditory cortex using rabbits anaesthetized with Dial (see also Neal *et al.*, 1968). In accord with previous findings, electrical stimulation of the somato-sensory, visual and reticular pathways increased cortical ACh release, and upon stimulation of the ipsilateral medial geniculate body ACh release was greatest from the auditory cortex (Fig. 6.14). Also, the

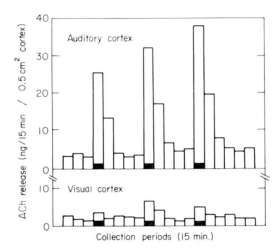

FIG. 6.14. Release of ACh from left auditory and left visual cortex during stimulation of the ipsilateral medial geniculate body of rabbits anaesthetized with "Dial". 15-min. periods of electrical stimulation at 10/s (1 ms duration) are indicated by horizontal bars. Reproduced with permission from Hemsworth and Mitchell (1969).

evoked release of ACh from auditory cortex was shown: (1) to be frequency dependent, as was found for ACh release from the visual cortex (Collier and Mitchell, 1966); (2) to require $Ca^{2+}$ (Fig. 6.15; see also, Randić and Padjen, 1967); (3) to be inhibited by high concentrations of $Mg^{2+}$.

Phillis (1968a) compared the resting and evoked release of ACh from several areas of the cat cortex using various anaesthetic agents. Resting ACh release occurred to a greater extent from somato-sensory areas of the cortex than from visual, auditory or parietal areas, and was greater in cats anaesthetized with diethyl ether, halothane or Dial than in those anaesthetized with pentobarbitone-$Na^+$ or chloralose. It was shown further that stimulation of a variety of peripheral afferent pathways produced comparable increases in ACh release from all cortical areas tested (Table 16). For example, in cats anaesthetized with diethyl ether, auditory and visual stimulation evoked a similar release of ACh from somato-sensory, auditory, visual and parietal cortices (Fig. 6.16). Similar effects were shown in chloralose-anaesthetized cats (Fig. 6.17), although chloralose has been shown to have an inhibitory action of ACh release (see e.g. MacIntosh and Oborin, 1953; Mitchell, 1963). Comparable increases in ACh release were produced by electrical stimulation of the reticular formation of the cortex. On the basis or these results, Phillis

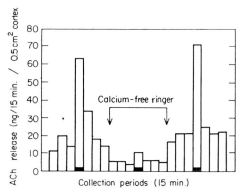

FIG. 6.15. Spontaneous and evoked release of ACh from the auditory cortex by stimulation of the ipsilateral medial geniculate body at 20/s (1 ms duration) in the absence and in the presence of $Ca^{2+}$. Periods of electrical stimulation are indicated by horizontal bars; "Dial"-anaesthetized rabbits. Reproduced with permission from Hemsworth and Mitchell (1969).

suggested that the reticulo-cortical system, rather than specific thalamo-cortical systems, is the major system involved in ACh release (see also Bartolini *et al.*, 1972). These results of Phillis (1968a), and those of Bartolini *et al.* (1972) which were obtained in un-anaesthetized cats transected at midpontine levels, are not in agreement with the hypothesis that specific cholinergic thalamo-cortical pathways exist (Collier and Mitchell, 1966, 1967; Brownlee and Mitchell, 1968; Hemsworth and Mitchell, 1969). However, in recent iontophoretic studies (Stone, 1972) it was shown that ACh and muscarinic agonists exerted excitatory actions, especially in cells of the somato-sensory cortex, which responded to specific thalamic stimulation. This finding indicated that ACh might serve as an excitatory transmitter in a specific thalamo-cortical pathway, and therefore lends some support to the contention of Mitchell and co-workers. It seems possible that differences in the duration of the applied stimuli and/or in the type of anaesthetic (and level of anaesthesia) used may be at the basis of this discrepancy (see also §2.1 and Chapter 5). In any case, it remains possible that the evoked increases in ACh collectability which have been shown may not be related to "physiological" transmitter release. The various stimuli used to increase ACh collectability could have affected AChE or ChAc activities or may have produced increases in the utilization of ACh in non-transmitter systems,

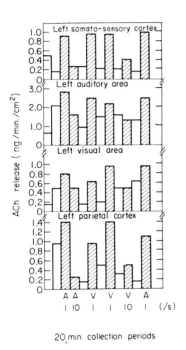

Fig. 6.16. Rates of release of ACh from areas of cat cortex during auditory (A) and visual (V) stimulation. The cat was anaesthetized with diethyl ether. Reproduced with permission from Phillis (1968a).

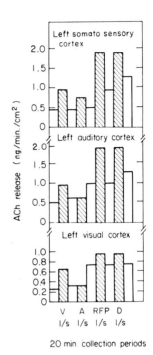

Fig. 6.17. A comparison of the effects of visual (V), auditory (A), contralateral forepaw (RFP) and direct cortical (D) stimulation on the rate of release of ACh from primary cortical areas of a cat anaesthetized with chloralose. Reproduced with permission from Phillis (1968a).

and these changes may have occurred to different extents in the various areas of the cortex. The results of Phillis (1968a) have indicated further that resting ACh release occurs to a rather similar extent from several areas of the cortex when Dial is compared with halothane. However, Dudar and Szerb (1969) found that ACh release was about five times greater with Dial than with halothane-$N_2O$. It seems, as suggested by Dudar and Szerb (1969), that their use of halothane together with $N_2O$

TABLE 16. Mean percentage increase in rate of release of ACh[a] induced by various modes of stimulation in cats anaesthetized with pentobarbitone Na$^+$. Reproduced with permission from Phillis (1968a).

| Cortical area | Left forepaw | Left hindpaw | Left facial | Auditory | Visual | Reticular formation | Direct cortical[c] |
|---|---|---|---|---|---|---|---|
| Right somato-sensory | 230(25–650)[b] | 120(20–260) | 170(30–280) | 100(20–170) | 160(40–220) | — | 120(80–170) |
| Left somato-sensory | 250(0–650) | 50(0–100) | 190(30–350) | 110(0–300) | 100(10–180) | 180(40–320) | 140(100–210) |
| Auditory | 320(80–650) | — | 130(10–250) | 85(0–190) | 120(30–200) | 210(80–320) | 100(50–160) |
| Visual | 90(25–150) | — | 70(20–130) | 80(65–100) | 110(30–200) | 70(30–160) | 30(10–60) |
| Parietal | 30(5–60) | — | — | — | — | — | — |

[a] Rates of release immediately before and after stimulation were used to calculate baselines for these figures.

[b] Ranges.

[c] Stimulation of left somato-sensory cortex within the cup. ACh release was simultaneously determined.

could have produced deeper anaesthesia than that produced by halo-thane, alone, and that this could have caused this discrepancy (see MacIntosh and Oborin, 1953; Mitchell, 1963). But, the different doses of Dial used (i.e. 0·6 mg/kg by Phillis and 0·8 mg/kg by Dudar and Szerb) could also have accounted for much of this difference (Phillis, 1972; personal communication).

As would be expected, systemic injections of convulsant drugs, such as metrazol, picrotoxin, and strychnine, also cause increases in cortical

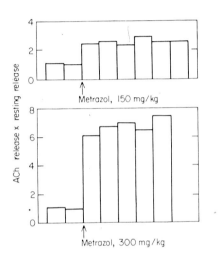

Fig. 6.18. Effect of metrazol (leptazol; 150 and 300 mg/kg) on the mean ACh release from the cerebral cortex (8 rats anaesthetized with "Dial"). Each block represents a 30 min. collection period. EEG showed convulsive discharges which coincided with the increased collectability of ACh. Reproduced with permission from Hemsworth and Neal (1968).

ACh release which correlate with activated EEG activity (Mitchell, 1963; Hemsworth and Neal, 1968; Szerb *et al.*, 1970; Figs 6.18–6.20). Szerb *et al.*, (1970) showed that the increase in cortical ACh release caused by picrotoxin injections in cats was reflected by a decrease in the ACh content of the cortex (Fig. 6.19), and that these effects of picrotoxin were increased by prior treatment of the animals with atropine (Fig. 6.20). A further interesting finding was obtained in un-anaesthetized pre-trigeminally-sectioned cats; i.e. topically-applied atropine (1 μg/ml) increased cortical ACh release while not affecting cortical ACh content (Szerb *et al.*, 1970; Fig. 6.21). This finding led to studies on the nature of atropine-induced ACh release in cerebral cortical slices in which it was shown that the enhancing effect of atropine on the *in vivo* release of ACh might be explained, in part, by its effect of overcoming the

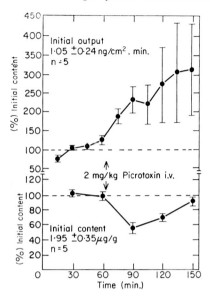

FIG. 6.19. The effects of intravenous injection of picrotoxin (2 mg/kg) on cortical ACh output and content in cats anaesthetized with "Dial". Reproduced with permission from Szerb *et al.*, (1970).

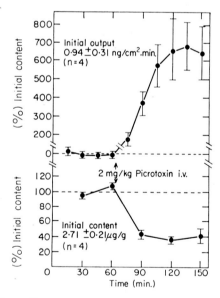

FIG. 6.20. The effects of intravenous injections of picrotoxin (2 mg/kg) on cortical ACh output and content in cats anaesthetized with "Dial" and pretreated with atropine (1 mg/kg, i.v.) 90 min. before starting experiments. Reproduced with permission from Szerb *et al.*, (1970).

reduction in ACh release caused by anti-ChE agents, such as eserine (Szerb and Somogyi, 1973). It is also well known that sympathomimetic amines, such as amphetamines, cause central cholinergic activation (e.g. White and Daigneault, 1959; Arnfred and Randrup, 1968). Increases in ACh release from the cortex also occurred after systemic administration of amphetamine to cats or rats (Pepeu and Bartolini, 1968; Hemsworth and Neal, 1968; Fig. 6.22; see also §2.5), and this release of ACh

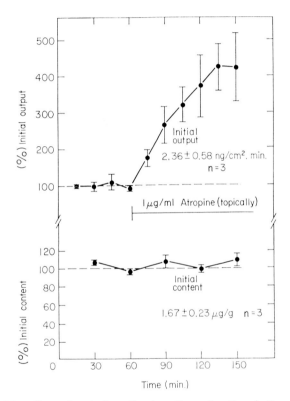

Fig. 6.21. The effects of topical application of atropine (1 μg/ml) on cortical ACh output and content in pre-trigeminally-sectioned, im-anaesthetized cats. Reproduced with permission from Szerb *et al.*, (1970).

was correlated with an increase in blood pressure and with EEG activation and seemed to involve the reticulo-cortical arousal system (Bradley and Elkes, 1957; White and Daigneault, 1959). Control experiments indicated that the effect on blood pressure could not have accounted for the increased ACh release caused by amphetamine (Pepeu and Bartolini, 1968). Amphetamine also produced an increase in ACh release which was associated with EEG activation in cats transected at the pre-collicular level while electrical stimulation of the midbrain in this preparation had no effect on either ACh release or the EEG (Deffenu *et al.*, 1970). In a more recent study, Nistri *et al.*, (1972) demonstrated, also in the cat, that the increase in ACh release, but not the EEG activation, produced by amphetamine was prevented by electro-coagulation of the septum (see also §5.3). Septal lesions also prevented amphetamine-induced increases in ACh release in the rat (Pepeu, 1972).

Administration of angiotensin can cause EEG arousal in cats (Uchikawa, 1964). In "encephale isolé" cats, Elie and Panisset (1970) showed

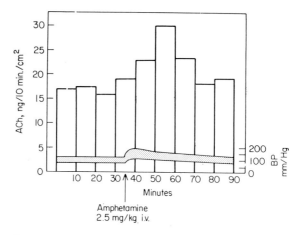

Fig. 6.22. Effects of an intravenous injection of amphetamine (2·5 mg/kg) on cortical ACh output and blood pressure in a cat transected at the mid-pontine, pre-trigeminal level. Reproduced with permission from Pepeu and Bartolini (1968).

that locally-applied angiotensin ($10^{-9}$ M) increased ACh release from the parietal cortex. Intra-cortically-administered angiotensin (1 ng/ 0·1 $\mu$l; 1 mm deep) also increased markedly the output of ACh. Although the mechanism of this effect of angiotensin remains unknown, these findings add support to the idea that ACh is involved in arousal. Centrally-active analgesics such as morphine (0·1, 1·0 and 5·0 mg/kg, i.v.) and levallorphan (0·1 and 1·0 mg/kg, i.v.) reduced ACh release from different regions of cat cortex; the reduction by morphine could be reversed by 5 mg/kg levallorphan (Jhamandas *et al.*, 1970, 1971). Narcotic antagonists (naloxone and nalorphine) also antagonized the reduction of ACh release caused by morphine. These studies indicated that the opiates may act by blocking some part of the arousal response (see also Polak, 1965; Beani *et al.*, 1968). EEG synchronization and general sedation have also been shown to accompany morphine-induced depression of cortical ACh release in conscious rabbits (Beani *et al.*, 1968; Fig. 6.23).

The writer does not believe that ACh is the only pharmacologically-active substance released from the cortex by the various stimuli which produce EEG, or behavioural, arousal. This notion finds some support in the recent results of Jasper and Koyama (1967, 1968, 1969) which indi-cated that the excitatory amino acid, glutamate, can also be released by electrical stimulation of the MRF in "encephale isolé" cats. Reticular stim-ulation also caused increases in aspartate, glycine and taurine release, and

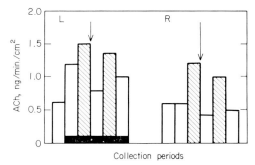

FIG. 6.23. Release of ACh into fluid of left (L) and right (R) epidural cups in a conscious rabbit, 5 days after surgery. Vertical bars indicate 30 min. collection periods; ■ indicates the application of atropine ($4 \times 10^{-7}$ g/ml); hatched bars indicate electrical stimulation of an ear. At the ↓, 5 mg/kg morphine was intravenously injected. Reproduced with permission from Beani *et al.*, (1968).

the release of glutamate was much greater than that of ACh (Fig. 6.24). Since electrical stimulation of mesial thalamic areas increased ACh release without altering glutamate release in the studies of Jasper and Koyama, it was suggested that different pathways might be involved in the release of ACh and glutamate. It seems possible, therefore, that ACh might be involved in pathways of EEG arousal as well as in those re-sponsible for cortical recruiting responses, but that glutamate may be involved only in the arousal mechanism. These findings could also mean that ACh and glutamate pathways are in overlap in the mesencephalon, but not in the thalamus (Jasper and Koyama, 1969). These results have provided further support for the concept that the ACh collected at the cortical surface can be due to activation of at least two different afferent pathways (see also Collier and Mitchell, 1966, 1967). A criterion which may be helpful in establishing the identity of transmitter substances may be to consider the candidate substances on the basis of their pharmaco-logical potencies in a given area of the CNS; thus, both ACh and gluta-mate would qualify for roles in the arousal mechanism. Also, the transmitter used in a given central pathway should depend not only on its release from pre-synaptic terminals but also on the specific receptor properties of the post-synaptic membranes involved.

With regard to the ionic mechanisms involved in the cortical release of ACh, it has been shown that either omission of $Ca^{2+}$ or increased $Mg^{2+}$ in perfusion fluids reduces both spontaneous and evoked release in Dial-anaesthetized cats or rabbits (Randić and Padjen, 1967; Hemsworth and Mitchell, 1969; see Fig. 6.15). These results provide some

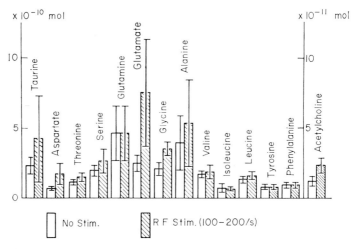

FIG. 6.24. Rates of release of amino acids ("acidic and neutral series") and ACh at rest and during electrical stimulation of the mesencephalic reticular formation (MRF) in "encephal isolé" preparations (6 cats). □ represent collections made during periods of rest, characterized by slow-wave sleep; ▨ represent collections made during stimulation of the MRF at 100–200/s (means ± S.E.M.). Glutamate acid, aspartate acid, taurine, glycine and ACh were increased significantly by MRF stimulation. Reproduced with permission from Jasper and Koyama (1969).

support for the idea that the release of ACh in the cortex may be similar to that which occurs at the neuromuscular junction (e.g. del Castillo and Katz, 1954, 1956; Hubbard, 1961; Hubbard *et al.*, 1968). In other experiments, performed on cats under Dial anaesthesia, the presence of tetrodotoxin (TTX; 2–10 $\mu$g/ml) in perfusion fluids caused a significant reduction in the resting rate of ACh release from the cortex, which may have been due to a blocking effect of TTX on action potentials in cholinergic neurones (Dudar and Szerb, 1969; Bjegović *et al.*, 1969; see Fig. 6.25). Also, atropine, applied after TTX, did not cause an increase in ACh release which indicated that cortical ACh release by atropine may depend on continuous neural activity (Dudar and Szerb, 1969).

Hence, it seems likely that atropine might increase the collectability of a physiologically-active transmitter pool of ACh. Perfusion of the cortical surface with $Na^+$-free Ringer's solution (i.e. Ringer's in which all $Na^+$ was substituted by $Li^+$) blocked ACh release evoked by stimulation of the contralateral forepaw in cats, while not affecting resting release Bjegović and Randić, 1971). Since TTX has been shown to prevent increases in $Na^+$ conductance (Kao, 1966) and since $Li^+$ is not pumped from spinal motoneurones as readily as $Na^+$ (Araki *et al.*, 1965), it seems likely, when considering these findings together with those outlined above, that cortical ACh release may depend on the inward transport

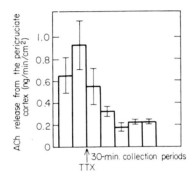

FIG. 6.25. Effect of tetrodotoxin (*TTX*) on the release of ACh from the pericruciate cortex in cats anaesthetized with "Dial" (means ± standard deviations; n = 4). *TTX* ($2 \times 10^{-6}$ g/ml) was applied locally for 150 min. (*arrow*). Reproduced with permission from Bjegović *et al.* (1969).

of $Na^+$ (see Birks, 1963; Narahashi *et al.*, 1964). These findings concerning the ionic basis of ACh release, along with the findings that atropine does not increase ACh release in the absence of neural activity (nervous impulses) and that TTX may reduce ACh release by blocking action potentials in cholinergic neurones (Dudar and Szerb, 1969), provide good evidence that the ACh collected from the surface of the cortex may be released as a transmitter. The similarities which have been found between cortical and neuromuscular mechanisms add further strength to this view.

From the information provided above, it certainly seems possible that ACh release is involved in mechanisms of cortical activation. However, one might ask about the relevancy of these observations to the mechanisms of cortical activation or depression which occur in the awake, behaving animal, or about ACh release which may occur in response to traumatic brain injury. Studies on ACh release have been conducted in awake animals and correlate rather well with those performed with anaesthetized or lesioned animals. In early experiments it was shown that pentobarbital and other anaesthetics affected the ACh content of the brain; i.e. the greater the depth of anaesthesia, within certain limits, the higher the content of cerebral ACh (Tobias *et al.*, 1946; Richter and

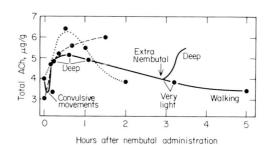

Hours after nembutal administration

FIG. 6.26. Total ACh content of rat brain at various times after equal intra-peritoneal injections of pentobarbital (Nembutal). Each curve represents results with a group of similar rats treated with Nembutal at the same time. Reproduced with permission from Elliott *et al.* (1950).

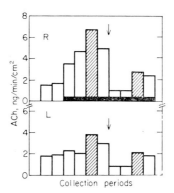

Collection periods

FIG. 6.27. Release of ACh into fluid of right (R) and left (L) epidural cups in a conscious rabbit, 20 h after implantation of the cups. *Veritcal bars* indicate 30 min. collection periods; *solid bar* indicates the application of atropine ($4 \times 10^{-7}$ g/ml); *hatched bars* indicate electrical stimulation of an ear. At the *arrow*, 20 mg/kg pento-barbital was intravenously injected. Reproduced with permission from Beani *et al.* (1968).

Crossland, 1949; Elliott *et al.*, 1950; Crossland and Merrick, 1954; see Fig. 6.26). Later, Collier and Mitchell (1967) showed further that pento-barbital produced changes in ACh release from the cerebral cortex in conscious rabbits which reflected the changes in brain ACh content shown by previous workers (Fig. 6.13). Studies by Beani *et al.*, (1968) indicated that both topically-administered atropine and electrical stimulation of the ear cause increases in ACh release to fluid in epidural cups in conscious rabbits, and that these increases in ACh release could be prevented by pentobarbital (Fig. 6.27) or morphine (Fig. 6.23) and enhanced by amphetamine. With regard to experimental brain injury, Metz (1971b) has shown that ACh release from the cerebral cortex of

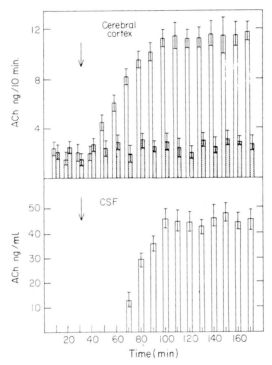

FIG. 6.28. *Upper graph:* Release of ACh from the cerebral cortex of a dog after a blow (*at arrow*) to the cortical surface (*white bars*); the non-traumatized contralateral side is represented by *stippled bars. Lower graph:* Simultaneous measurement of the ACh content of the CSF. Vertical lines at the tops of the bars indicate S.E.M. Reproduced from Metz (1971b), with permission from the editors of *Journal of Neurosurgery.*

anaesthetized dogs was increased significantly when these animals were subjected to a blow to the cortical surface (Figs 6.28 and 6.29). Also, ACh was present in the CSF after the injury (Fig. 6.28), and exposure of the animals to hypercapnia (12 % $CO_2$) increased further the ACh release from the non-traumatized side while not affecting the traumatized side (Fig. 6.29). It was suggested that ACh may be released from damaged cells during brain injury. In this regard, it seems noteworthy that Tower and MacEachern (1949a, b), in their studies on humans, could detect ACh in the CSF only in some epileptics and craniocerebral trauma patients.

Although these results seem to provide evidence that cortical ACh release is associated with changes in behavioural as well as EEG arousal, the effects of psychoactive drugs on these parameters are not predictable (see Table 17), and hence a number of problems remain to be solved.

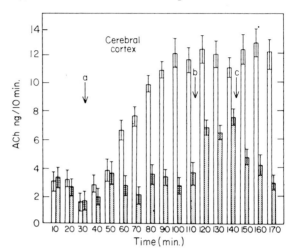

Fig. 6.29. Release of ACh from dog cerebral cortex after a blow to its surface (at arrow *a*) and during hypercapnia (between arrows *b* and *c*). *White bars* represent the traumatized side; *stippled bars* represent the non-traumatized contralateral side. Vertical lines indicate S.E.M. Reproduced with permission from the editors of *Journal of Neurosurgery;* data of Metz (1971b).

Table 17. Effects of intravenous injections of some drugs on cortical ACh release, electrocorticogram and behaviour in rabbits. Reproduced with permission from Beani *et al.* (1968).

| Drug | Dose (mg/kg) | ACh release | Effect on electrocorticogram | Behaviour |
|---|---|---|---|---|
| Pentobarbital | 20 | Decrease | Synchronization | Anaesthesia |
| Amphetamine | 2 | Increase | Desynchronization | Excitement |
| Morphine | 5 | Decrease | Synchronization | Sedation |
| Atropine | 10 | Increase | Synchronization | No change |
| Chlorpromazine | 4 | No effect | Synchronization | Akinesia and indifference |

In recent experiments with freely-moving cats, Jasper and Tessier (1971) showed that cortical ACh release increased during paradoxical (r.e.m.) sleep and that this increase approximated to that which occurred during the waking state. These findings indicated that ACh release may be correlated to a greater extent with electro-cortical activity than with behavioural responsiveness. Perhaps the major problem which remains is related to the findings that atropine can cause EEG synchronization and increased ACh release with no dramatic changes in gross behaviour (see also Chapters 2 and 5; see above). However, it seems to be well established that atropine exerts major effects on operant behaviour (learning) and perhaps on memory (see Chapter 5, especially §§5.3 and 5.4). The effects of atropine on the EEG and on ACh release might be explained by its occupation of excitatory muscarinic receptors and by its preventative action on ACh re-uptake, respectively. The increased release of ACh produced by atropine may occur by its action of preventing a negative-feedback effect of extracellular ACh on pre-synaptic terminals (e.g. Szerb, 1967; Dudar and Szerb, 1969). However, its effects on behaviour which parallel these changes (see Chapter 5) might only be explained by postulating a series of different mechanisms operating at various levels of the neuraxis.

With regard to the apparent paradoxical effects of atropine on EEG and ACh release, it seems possible that part of the effect of atropine on ACh release *in vivo* may be due to its action of reducing the depressant effect which ChE inhibition causes on ACh release, and therefore, much of the observed effect of atropine on ACh release might not occur in normal animals in which ChE is not inhibited (Szerb, 1972, personal communication; see also Szerb *et al.*, 1970; Szerb and Somogyi, 1973). It has also been suggested recently that the atropine-induced increase in ACh release from the cortex may be due to an excess of muscarinic inhibitory over excitatory synapses in the cortex (Stone, 1972). With further regard to the effects of atropine and scopolamine on behaviour, it should be noted that marked species differences seem to exist. For instance, it is well known that operant behaviours are affected by atropine in rats and that atropine, in large doses produces dramatic behavioural changes in man, but both atropine (White *et al.*, 1961) and scopolamine (Méhes, 1929, White *et al.*, 1961) do not produce marked changes in gross behaviour in rabbits, even when administered in large doses (see also Beani *et al.*, 1968). White and Rudolph (1968) suggested that the cortical and subcortical actions of these agents may differ between rabbits and other species. However, Giarman and Pepeu (1962) found that atropine injections decreased markedly brain ACh in rats while exerting no obvious effects on their gross behaviour. In a recent study it has been shown that lower intravenous doses of atropine were needed to increase cortical ACh release than to enhance motor activity in rats (Aquilonius *et al.*, 1972), which indicated that the effect of atropine on ACh release was related to cortical sites while that on motor behaviour was subserved by sub-cortical mechanisms.

*B. Caudate Nucleus, Thalamus, Hypothalamus and Mesencephalon*

It is well known that the caudate nucleus, thalamus, hypothalamus and mesencephalon all contain large amounts of ACh, ChAc, and AChE (e.g. MacIntosh, 1941; Feldberg and Vogt, 1948; Hebb and Silver, 1956; Krnjević and Silver, 1965; see Figs 2.15–2.18, 3.4–3.7, 4.6 and 4.7). Therefore, it seems reasonable to suppose that ACh may be a transmitter in these regions. The release of ACh from the caudate nucleus (and other structures) has been studied by perfusing ventricular spaces (Bhattacharya and Feldberg, 1957) and with push-pull cannulae

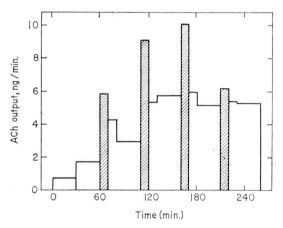

Time (min.)

Fig. 6.30. Collectability of ACh from the cerebral ventricles of a cat during perfusion with neostigmine, 1/50 000. *Hatched bars* indicate periods of electrical stimulation of the caudate nucleus. Cats were anaesthetized with chloralose. Reproduced with permission from Beleslin *et al.*, (1965).

(Gaddum, 1961); ACh release from the thalamus, hypothalamus and mesencephalon was studied using push-pull cannulae. Upon perfusion of the brains of chloralose-anaesthetized cats from lateral ventricle to aqueduct, in the presence of neostigmine, the ACh collected was presumably derived mainly from the caudate nucleus (Bhattacharya and Feldberg, 1958a, b; Beleslin *et al.*, 1964). About four times as much ACh was released by perfusion with neostigmine than with eserine or DFP (Bhattacharya and Feldberg, 1957). ACh release was reduced by addition of morphine or chloralose to perfusion fluids (Beleslin and Polak, 1965) and increased by intravenous injections of metrazol or strychnine (Beleslin *et al.*, 1965). Increases in the release of ACh were also produced by direct electrical stimulation of the caudate nucleus (Mitchell and Szerb, 1962; Beleslin *et al.*, 1965; Fig. 6.30). ACh release from the caudate nucleus was further potentiated by hyoscine given after metrazol (leptazol), and by metrazol given after hyoscine (Fig. 6.31), which indicated that the actions of these agents on ACh release might involve different mechanisms (see Polak, 1965). Using push-pull cannulae, McLennan (1964) found that an increase in ACh release from the caudate nucleus of pentobarbital-anaesthetized cats could be produced by low-frequency stimulation of the nucleus ventralis anterior

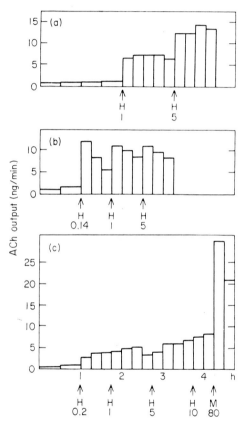

Fig. 6.31. ACh release in successive 30 and 15 min. samples collected from the cerebral ventricles perfused with solution containing neostigmine (1/50 000) in three anaesthetized cats. At arrows marked *H* or *M*, intravenous injections of hyoscine or metrazol) were administered; figures below letters refer to the doses in mg/kg. Reproduced with permission from Polak (1965).

(VA) of the thalamus. Since activation of VA affected the caudate nucleus, McLennan suggested that the final synapse in the VA-caudate pathway may be cholinergic. In more recent studies, it was shown, in cats, using either acutely- or chronically-implanted push-pull cannulae, that injection of chlorpromazine (10 mg/kg, i.v.) caused a marked increase in ACh release from the caudate nucleus which was abolished by apomorphine (10 mg/kg, i.v.) administered 1 h after the chlorpromazine (Stadler *et al.*, 1973). Phillis *et al.* (1968) studied ACh release, in the presence of neostigmine, from the thalami of cats anaesthetized with pentobarbitone or thiopentone-plus-$N_2O$, $O_2$ and methoxyflurane. Using push-pull cannulae, it was shown that resting ACh release occurred from both dorsal and ventro-basal nuclei. Photic, reticular

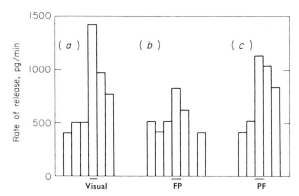

Fig. 6.32. Histograms showing the release of ACh from the ventro-basal thalamic complex in three anaesthetized cats, before, during and after stimulation (see text for anaesthetics). Each division of the abscissa represents one 10-min. collection period. (A) effect of visual stimulation (1/s); (B) effect of contralateral forepaw stimulation (1/s); (C) effect of stimulating the mesencephalic reticular formation (2/s). The positions of stimulating electrodes were histologically verified. Reproduced with permission from Phillis *et al.*, (1968).

and limb stimulations increased the release of ACh from ventro-basal nuclei (Fig. 6.32). It was suggested that the effects of photic and limb stimulations might be due to activation of the non-specific reticulocortical pathway and that the ACh release from the dorsal thalamus might be related to inhibitory cholinergic pathways (see e.g. McCance *et al.*, 1968). The spontaneous release of ACh has also been demonstrated in the thalamus, hypothalamus and superior colliculus of the unanaesthetized monkey (Myers and Beleslin, 1970; Beleslin and Myers, 1970).

## C. Medulla

Abundant evidence exists to support the contention that central respiratory reflexes may involve cholinergic mechanisms (see e.g. Metz, 1956, 1958, 1961, 1962, and §4.1), and some cells of the medulla are cholinoceptive (e.g. Bradley and Wolstencroft, 1962, 1965; Salmoiraghi and Steiner, 1963; Bradley *et al.*, 1966). But, the question of whether or not ACh plays a major role in the function of medullary neurones remains unanswered (Gessell and Hansen, 1945; Metz, 1961, 1962, 1964; Salmoiraghi and Steiner, 1963). Therefore, Metz (1966) studied, using push-pull cannulae, the resting release of ACh from the medulla and

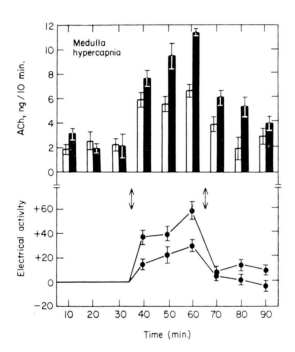

Fig. 6.33. Release of ACh from the medulla and correlated electrical activity of the medulla, before, during and after exposure of dogs to hypercapnia ($12\%$ $CO_2$). *Clear* and *solid bars* indicate, respectively, release from "non-respiratory-responsive" areas and "respiratory-responsive" areas; *upper* and *lower curves* represent, respectively, the mean integrated electrical activities of these two areas. Dogs were exposed to hypercapnia during the time indicated by the arrows. Resting electrical activity is set to 0 (means $\pm$ S.E.M.; 28 dogs). Dogs were anaesthetized with morphine sulphate plus urethane (2·5 mg/kg and 1 g/kg, respectively). Reproduced from Metz (1971a), with permission from the editors of *Canadian Journal of Physiology and Pharmacology*.

cerebral cortex in dogs anaesthetized with morphine-$SO_4$, followed by urethane. Hypercapnia ($12\%$ $CO_2$) increased significantly the release of ACh to perfusion fluids containing sarin from both medulla and cortex; effects of hypercapnia-plus-hypoxia ($12\%$ $CO_2 + 8\%$ $O_2$) were similar to those of hypercapnia; hypoxia ($8\%$ $O_2$) had no effect. Increases in ACh release caused by hypercapnia were more pronounced in "respiratory responsive areas" than in "non-respiratory responsive

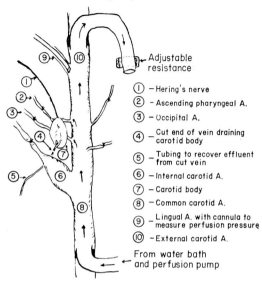

Adjustable
resistance

① – Hering's nerve
② – Ascending pharyngeal A.
③ – Occipital A.
④ – Cut end of vein draining
     carotid body
⑤ – Tubing to recover effluent
     from cut vein
⑥ – Internal carotid A.
⑦ – Carotid body
⑧ – Common carotid A.
⑨ – Lingual A. with cannula to
     measure perfusion pressure
⑩ – External carotid A.

From water bath
and perfusion pump

FIG. 6.34. Schematic drawing of perfusion of the isolated carotid body. Reproduced from Metz (1969), with permission from the editors of *Respiration Physiology*.

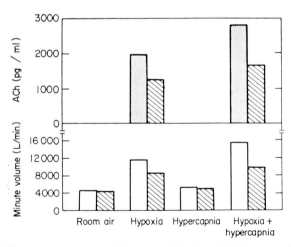

FIG. 6.35. Effects of perfusion of the carotid body with blood equilibrated with room air, low $O_2$, high $CO_2$, or low $O_2$ + high $CO_2$, on the minute volume of spontaneous respiratory responses and on the ACh content of the venous effluent from the carotid body. *White bars*, minute volume in 27 dogs; *black bars*, significant recovery of ACh in venous effluent during hypoxia (16 dogs) and hypoxia + hypercapnia (17 dogs); *hatched bars*, same animals after perfusion with solution containing HC-3 $(2 \times 10^{-4}$ M$)$. Twenty-seven dogs in minute volume data; significant recovery of ACh in 7 of the dogs during hypoxia, and in 8 of the dogs during hypoxia + hypercapnia. Reproduced from Metz (1969), with permission from the editors of *Respiration Physiology*.

areas" of the medullary reticular formation. In further studies it was shown that the increase in ACh release caused by hypercapnia correlated well with electrical activity in these areas (Metz, 1971a; Fig. 6.33), and that hypoxia or hypoxia + hypercapnia also caused a release of ACh from the isolated carotid body (which is involved in both respiratory and blood pressure control) in dogs (Metz, 1969; Figs 6.34 and 6.35). The evidence presented indicates that ACh may be involved in the central control of respiration (see also §4.1). However, it is noteworthy

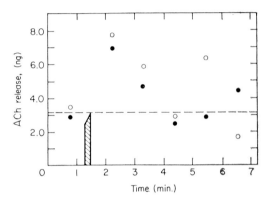

FIG. 6.36. Post-tetanic potentiation of ACh relaase to fluid used to perfuse the vascular supply of cat spinal cord. *Open* and *filled circles* represent data from 2 cats. Each point represents the amount of ACh recovered from 1 min. samples collected successively during stimulation of peripheral nerves at 5/second. Nerves were stimulated at 500/s for 10 s during the time indicated by the hatched bar; perfusion was begun at zero time. Reproduced with permission from Kuno and Rudomin (1966).

that the use of morphine could have reduced ACh release from the medulla in these studies (see e.g. Beleslin and Polak, 1965; Beani *et al.*, 1968; Jhamandas *et al.*, 1971).

### D. *Spinal Cord*

Considerable evidence exists for a transmitter role of ACh at certain spinal cord synapses (see e.g. Feldberg, 1945, 1950; Eccles, 1964, 1969; Phillis, 1970; Section 3.1), and a number of studies about ACh release from the spinal cord have been reported. Bülbring and Burn (1941) showed that stimulation of the sciatic nerve in dogs liberated a substance with ACh-like activity from the spinal cord to eserinized perfusion media. Later, Angelucci (1956) demonstrated that reflex activity in the frog (produced by hind-limb stimulation) caused several substances to be released from the spinal cord, one of which possessed ACh-like activity on eserinized leech muscle (see also Ramwell *et al.*, 1966). In studies with isolated frog spinal cord, Mitchell and Phillis (1962) showed that ACh was released continuously in the presence of antiChE agents, and that its rate of release was increased by antidromic stimulation of ventral roots, but not by stimulation of the spinal cord, itself, or of dorsal roots (Table 18). It was suggested that ACh was released mainly at axon collateral-"Renshaw" cell synapses, but that some ACh could have come from the ventral roots, themselves. Confirmation that ACh is released from motoneuronal axon collaterals was provided by Kuno and Rudomin (1966), who showed, by perfusing the vascular supply of cat lumbosacral cord (in the presence of eserine), that ACh release could be increased by stimulating sciatic or femoral nerves. It was shown further that both the collectability of ACh and Renshaw cell discharges were reduced by stimulation at frequencies greater than 10/second. Post-tetanic potentiation, which apparently indicates an enchancement of Renshaw cell activity (Eccles *et al.*, 1954), also produced increases in ACh release from the cord (Fig. 6.36). Kuno and Rudomin concluded that motoneuronal collateral-Renshaw cell synapses might have been the site of ACh release. Since part of ACh activity collected in studies by Bülbring and Burn (1941) and by Kuno and Rudomin (1966) could have been due to leakage from paravertebral muscles, it seems pertinent to mention that a method has been described which allows perfusion of the intermeningeal spaces of the spinal cord (Edery and Levinger, 1971).

TABLE 18. The spontaneous release of ACh from the frog spinal cord and the changes observed during electrical stimulation. Reproduced with permission from Mitchell and Phillis (1962).

| Maximal stimulation of: | Frequency of stimulation (stim/s) | Number of experiments | Average spontaneous release[a] (*p*-mol/15 min./ hemisected cord) | % Change during stimulation[b] |
|---|---|---|---|---|
| Dorsal roots | 1 | 6 | 6·5 | −13 |
|  | 4 | 4 | 9·0 | +10 |
| Ventral roots | 1 | 4 | 5·5 | +52 |
|  | 4 | 19 | 5·5 | +93 |
|  | 20 | 5 | 4·5 | +132 |
| Spinal cord | 1 | 3 | 6·0 | −20 |
|  | 4 | 4 | 8·0 | −7 |

[a] These values represent the group average of the spontaneously-released ACh immediately before and after the period of stimulation.

[b] The values in this column represent the group average of the change in release during stimulation.

These workers confirmed earlier results on the release of ACh from cat spinal cord by sciatic stimulation and concluded that this release was from synapses between motoneuronal axon collaterals and Renshaw cells and from ventral roots, as suggested by previous workers (see above).

### 6.3 *In vitro* Studies

#### A. *Release of ACh from Brain Slices*

It has been long known that the synthesis and release of ACh occur in slices of cerebral cortex which are immersed in a suitable bathing medium, the rates of these processes being increased markedly by the

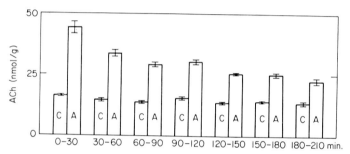

Fig. 6.37. ACh release (in n-mol/g, initial wet wt) from slices of rat cerebral cortex during seven successive 30 min. periods. Eight portions of slices were incubated simultaneously in separate vessels, four without (C) and four with (A) atropine ($3 \times 10^{-6}$ M). Means $\pm$ S.E.M.; n = 4. Reproduced with permission from Polak (1971a, b).

presence of high concentrations (e.g. about 25 mequiv/l) of $K^+$ in the medium (Mann *et al.*, 1939). Electrical stimulation of slices also increases their release of ACh (Rowsell, 1954), and in the presence of scopolamine a greater amount of ACh can be released by electrical stimulation (Bowers, 1967). Recently, it has been shown that both the synthesis and release of ACh in high-$K^+$ media can be increased further by adding atropine or other anti-muscarinic substances to the medium (Polak and Meeuws, 1966; Bertels-Meeuws and Polak, 1968; Polak, 1971a, b; Figs 6.37–6.40). Polak (1971a) concluded that the main action of atropine in slices might be to increase ACh release and that this increase in release could then cause increased ACh synthesis; i.e. by a negative feedback mechanism (see also Molenaar and Polak, 1970). In further experiments with slices of rat cerebral cortex, Bourdois *et al.*, (1971) showed that atropine at a concentration of $3 \times 10^{-7}$ M greatly enhanced ACh release evoked by electrical stimulation. It was also suggested that this action of atropine was likely to be due to a pre-synaptic action; i.e.

*Central Cholinergic Systems and Behaviour*

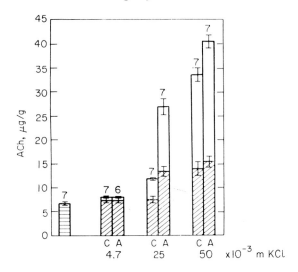

Fig. 6.38. Effects of atropine on the synthesis and release of ACh by slices of rat cerebral cortex bathed in media containing different concentrations of $K^+$. Slices were pre-incubated for 60 min. in medium containing 4·7 mequiv/l $K^+$ and then incubated for 60 min. in the presence of the various $K^+$ concentrations. Soman was used in all media. Incubation with ($A$) and without ($C$) atropine ($3 \times 10^{-6}$ M). ▤, ACh content at 0 min.; ▨, ACh content at 60 min; □, ACh released during 60 min.; means $\pm$ 2 $\times$ S.E.M.; numbers of observations indicated above each bar. Reproduced with permission from Bertels-Meeuws and Polak (1968).

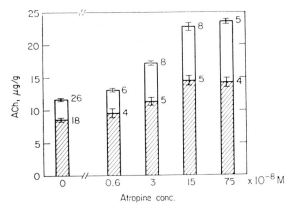

Fig. 6.39. Effects of atropine on the synthesis and release of ACh by slices of rat cerebral cortex. Slices were preincubated for 90 min. in medium containing 4·7 mequiv/l $K^+$ and then incubated for 60 min. in medium containing 25 mequiv/l $K^+$. Soman was used in all media. *Clear* and *hatched bars* represent, respectively, ACh release and content. Means $\pm$ S.E.M.; numbers of observations are indicated to the right of each bar. Reproduced with permission from Bertels-Meeuws and Polak (1968).

to its antagonism of a pre-synaptic inhibitory effect mediated by the released ACh.

In an attempt to define the mechanism by which atropine stimulated ACh release from slices, Polak (1971a, b) studied the interactions between atropine and two muscarinic agents (oxotremorine and metha-choline). Since his results indicated that the antagonism between atropine and these agents was "competitive", he suggested that the "ACh-releasing" effect of atropine might be due to its occupation of

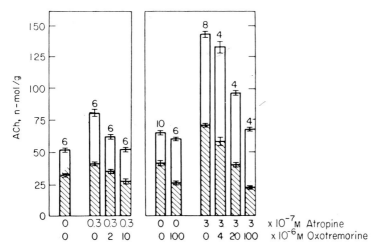

Fig. 6.40. ACh contents of rat cerebral cortex slices and incubation media after 60 min. incubation with and without atropine and oxotremorine. *Clear* and *hatched bars* represent, respectively, ACh in medium and ACh in slices; means ± S.E.M.; numbers of experiments above bars. ACh content is based upon initial wet weight of tissue. Reproduced with permission from Polak (1971a, b).

muscarinic receptors (see Fig. 6.40). The finding that atropine increased ACh release only in $K^+$-stimulated slices is in accord with earlier work (Bowers, 1967) in which it was shown that scopolamine increased ACh release only in electrically-stimulated slices. These findings shed light on the mechanism of action of atropine in the cerebral cortex, since they indicate that in order for atropine to cause ACh release the tissue must be activated. The mechanisms described above may be useful for explaining the increased release of ACh which is caused by atropine or atropine-like substances *in vivo* (e.g. Mitchell, 1963; Szerb, 1964; Polak, 1965; Celesia and Jasper, 1966; Bartolini and Pepeu, 1967; Dudar and Szerb, 1969). But, in more recent studies it has been shown, also in cortex slices, that the "ACh-releasing" effect of atropine may be due primarily to its action of preventing anti-ChE-induced decreases in ACh release

(Szerb and Somogyi, 1973). (In Polak's studies, the anti-ChE agent, soman (5 $\mu$M) was present in incubation media.) This finding may also be relevant in explaining the *in vivo* actions of atropine on ACh release since anti-ChE agents have been used in these release studies. It is also noteworthy that TTX did not block ACh release produced by atropine in slices (Polak, 1971a, b) as it did in *in vivo* experiments (Dudar and Szerb, 1969). However, these studies are not strictly comparable since

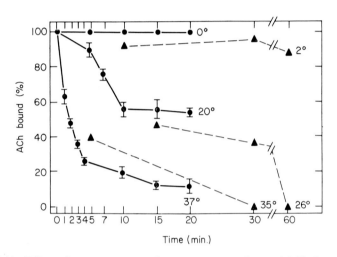

Fig. 6.41. Effect of temperature on the spontaneous release of ACh from isolated synaptic vesicles suspended in 0·4 M sucrose solution. Each point (●) an͏ bar represent the mean ± S.E.M. for at least 4 experiments. The zero point on the curve represents the amount of ACh initially bound to the vesicles and is defined as 100%. All other values are expressed as percentages of the zero time value. The average zero time value was 35 ± 3·5 *ng*/ml, which corresponds to a value of 61·3 *ng*/g of tissue. The curves at 2° and 26° C indicate the results obtained by Whittaker and Marchbanks (personal communication to Barker *et al.*, 1967); the curve at 35° C depicts data of Whittaker *et al.* (1964). Reproduced with permission from Barker *et al.* (1967).

with slices high K$^+$ concentrations had to be used to show the atropine-induced increase in ACh release, while in the *in vivo* studies the effect of atropine was easily shown in media containing normal K$^+$ concentrations. Other substances, such as Cobra venom lecithinase (Braganca and Quastel, 1952) and phospholipases A and C (Heilbronn, 1970), also cause a release of ACh from brain slices.

### B. *Release of ACh from Subcellular Particles*

Whittaker (1959) has discussed the effects which various ions, enzymes and physical treatments exert on the release and storage of ACh in synaptosomes (see also Marchbanks, 1969). Guth (1962) demonstrated that chlorpromazine prevents both the release and uptake of ACh by synaptosomes, and this agent also inhibits ACh binding to a synaptic vesicle fraction (Kuriyama *et al.*, 1968). Barker *et al.* (1967) studied the temperature-dependency of spontaneous ACh release from synaptic vesicles. It was found that after 20 min. of incubation at 0°C no ACh was released, but that appreciable release occurred at 20°C and at 37°C

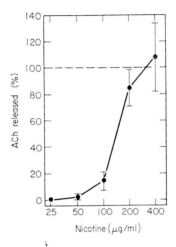

Fig. 6.42. Release of ACh from synaptic vesicles, prepared from rat cerebral cortex, by various concentrations of nicotine. Reproduced with permission from Chiou *et al.* (1970).

(Fig. 6.41). The absolute rate of release of ACh from the vesicles was proportional to the initial amount bound and release occurred in two phases, an initial rapid phase possibly being related to the surface, and a slower one to the interior, of the vesicles. This temperature-dependent release of ACh from synaptic vesicles can be stimulated by high $Na^+$ and low $K^+$ concentrations in the medium (Matsuda *et al.*, 1968). ATP and several nicotinic agents also can cause a release of endogenous ACh from synaptic vesicles prepared from cerebral cortex (Matsuda *et al.*, 1968; Chiou *et al.*, 1970; see Fig. 6.42).

### 6.4 Validity of Collection Methods

Hebb and Krnjević (1962) have discussed the diffusion of ACh which can occur into collecting cups placed on the exposed cerebral cortex in the presence of eserine. Evidence that this ACh this of parenchymal origin derives from the finding that no ACh has been detected in blood collected from superficial cortical veins (Mitchell, 1960). However, the release of

ACh measured by the "cup" method is subject to variation due to many factors which include: (1) depth and type of anaesthesia used; (2) tissue injury in the perfusion area; (3) type of anti-ChE agent used; (4) changes in blood and CSF pressure or compartmentation; (5) changes caused by applied stimuli (e.g. changes in the geometry of the cup-to-cortical surface relationship or changes in blood pressure caused by electrical stimulation). Although some investigators (e.g. Elie and Panisset, 1970) consider that the report by Collier and Murray-Brown validates the cup method, further more rigorously controlled experiments are necessary. For instance, if, in the above study, radioactive ACh had been applied topically to the surface of the cortex as was the radioactive urea which was used, perhaps no increase in the collectability of radioactive ACh would have been caused by electrical stimulation. This idea receives support from the recent study of Collier (1970) in which it was shown that direct electrical stimulation did not release radioactive ACh that had been allowed to diffuse into the cat's cerebral cortex, in the presence of DFP. It has also been suggested recently that the ACh collected from the cortical surface may be from a pool which has been more recently synthesized than that present in synaptosomal or vesicular fractions of the cortex (Chakrin *et al.*, 1972); this may be a non-transmitter pool of ACh. Studies performed using push-pull cannulae are subject to these same criticisms and, in addition, blood vessels are damaged during this procedure. Therefore, toxic substances present in blood, which do not penetrate into the brain under normal conditions, can enter the brain and affect the collectability of ACh. Ventricular perfusion systems are also subject to many of the above criticisms and, in addition, the substance must penetrate through the ependymal lining of the ventricles before it can be collected. Ventricular perfusion is a very indirect method for studying ACh release from the brain (see also §5.1, D).

### 6.5 The Nature of the Released Substance

It is particularly noteworthy that in most cases fluids used in perfusion (or "superfusion") studies have been analysed for their ACh contents using bioassay methods (e.g. leech muscle; frog rectus abdominus muscle; eviscerated cat's blood pressure; rat or guinea pig intestine; clam heart). Although some of these bioassay methods are quite sensitive to ACh, they cannot always be used to distinguish among the various substances present in fluids which possess "ACh-like" activity, and therefore, results presented in some reports may be subject to reinterpretation. A report by Hosein *et al.*, (1962) which indicated that the "ACh-like" activity in brain homogenates could be due largely to the presence of CoA esters of $\gamma$-butyrobetaine, crotonbetaine and carnitine, and to proprionylcholine and butyrycholine, stimulated Szerb (1963) to study the nature of the substances released to perfusion fluids. In Szerb's experiments, push-pull cannulae were implanted in cat somato-sensory cortex and "ACh-like" activity was released to fluid containing DFP by stimulation of the contralateral forepaw; the cats were anaes-thetized with Dial and injected with atropine. By parallel bioassay of the released material, he concluded that the activity was due to ACh, or a very similar ester. It should be noted that the substances used in this release experiment, as in other experiments of this type (e.g. DFP, atropine, Dial) could have influenced this assay system. Even though good agreement has been shown recently between bioassay and gas-chromatographic analyses of ACh in brain "extracts" (e.g. Stavinoha and Ryan, 1965; Holmstedt and Lundgren, 1966; Hanin, 1969), this has not been shown with "perfusates". Perhaps with the further develop-ment of methods based on gas-chromatography, mass fragmentography or fluorescence (Stavinoha and Ryan, 1965; Hammar *et al.*, 1968; Hanin, 1969; Campbell *et al.*, 1970; O'Neill and Sakimoto, 1970), better esti-mates of the amounts of "ACh-like" activity in perfusates which are due to ACh, itself, will be made. In a recent review, studies on the nature of the cholinomimetic activity of brain extracts have been discussed (Hebb and Morris, 1969).

# Chapter 7
# Conclusions

In the first six chapters of this monograph an attempt has been made to explain, in an interdisciplinary fashion, some of the central roles of cholinergic systems. It is only by continued effort along this line that the functional roles of central cholinergic systems will be correlated with the regulation of behaviour. In Chapter 1 the complexity of the problem at hand has been defined, in Chapters 2, 3 and 4, some of the more general roles of central cholinergic systems have been presented, in Chapter 5 an approach has been made to relate central cholinergic systems to complex behaviours, and in Chapter 6 the significant contributions derived from "release" studies have been described in some detail.

It should be noted that the data of previous investigators has been analysed in terms of the chemical theory of neurotransmission, and specifically, in terms of the cholinergic system. However, complex systems, such as arousal, sleep and wakefulness, homeostatic mechanisms, motivation, learning and memory cannot by explained simply in terms of a single postulated transmitter system, or in terms of transmitter theory, itself. Even if ACh is proven to be a transmitter that is involved in all of the complex behaviours of mammals, a complete description of these behaviours will require a knowledge of other central systems involved both in neurotransmission and in other mechanisms of nervous regulation and integration. It is necessary, therefore, to approach complex functional and behavioural systems by employing an interdisciplinary approach, and to strive for "molar" concepts of nervous function (see Hebb, 1949). This might be accomplished by manipulating the environment and/or nutrition of experimental animals and then analysing the resulting changes in brain and behaviour, or by studying animals in relation to maturation during which concomitant changes occur in brain and behaviour.

Perhaps the primary concept which has emerged from the analysis which has been carried out here, is that one can learn much about the CNS and its main expression, behaviour, by studying a proposed central transmitter system. The knowledge obtained about brain and behaviour in studies focused on central cholinergic mechanisms far outweighs the possible significance of such mechanisms in the regulation of central activity.

Much literature has accumulated which links environment, and especially early experience, to brain function and learning (see e.g. §5.4). However, only recently have biochemical and morphological studies been conducted, some on the cholinergic system, which provide evidence for a morphological basis of behaviour. The mammalian brain undergoes changes in its synaptic morphology and biochemistry, and hence, in its transmitter turnover and general metabolism, in response to changes in environment (see e.g. Chapter 5). By subjecting man or other animals to drastic changes in social environment (e.g. social isolation), behavioural disturbances, reflected as changes in emotionality and motivation, and hence in learning and memory, can be produced (see e.g. Bexton *et al.*, 1954; Heron, 1961; Reisen, 1966; Schweikart and Collins, 1966). Exposure of infant human beings or experimental animals to non-stimulating environments during critical periods of brain development can produce changes in their behaviour and in their learning abilities which are essentially irreversible (see e.g. Spitz, 1945; Hymovich, 1952; Bingham and Griffiths, 1952; Harlow and Harlow, 1962; Burns and Kimura, 1963; Mason, 1963; Welch, 1965; Harlow *et al.*, 1965, 1966; Sackett, 1968; Zubek, 1969; Prescott, 1971; see references in Morgan, 1973). It seems obvious from the data discussed in this monograph that central cholinergic systems are involved in these changes, which brings to mind once again the pioneering studies of Krech and coworkers in which it was shown that brain AChE activity changed as a function of environmental stimulation (see e.g. Bennett *et al.*, 1964; Rosenzweig and Leimann, 1968; Bennett and Rosenzweig, 1971).

It seems possible to study further the basis of behavioural regulation by making an interdisciplinary analysis of central cholinergic systems, or of any other system widely represented in the CNS. It is only when attempting to describe complex behaviours in terms of the actions of single cells that one runs into serious difficulty. Therefore, the analysis should perhaps be carried out at the level of discrete central structures, or better, discrete central pathways, in order to define, in a more general way, the underlying bases for behavioural change. In essence, this approach has been followed in many studies in which lesioning and direct injection techniques were employed, but, to date, systematic studies of the changes in regional biochemistry and in behaviour which can be produced by environmental or nutritional modification, or which occur during maturation, of animals, have not been conducted. Perhaps such studies will be carried out in the future.

# References

Abood, L. G. and Biel, J. H. (1962). Anticholinergic psychotomimetic agents. *Int. Rev. Neurobiol.* **4**, 217–273.

Abrahams, V. C., Koelle, G. B. and Smart, P. (1957). Histochemical demonstration of cholinesterases in the hypothalamus of the dog. *J. Physiol. (Lond.)* **139**, 137–144.

Abrahams, V. C. and Pickford, M. (1956). The effect of anticholinesterases injected into the supraoptic nuclei of chloralosed dogs on the release of the oxytocic factor of the posterior pituitary. *J. Physiol. (Lond.)* **133**, 330–333.

Adey, W. R., Segundo, J. P. and Livingston, R. B. (1957). Corticofugal influences on intrinsic brain stem conduction in cat and monkey. *J. Neurophysiol.* **20**, 1–16.

Albert, D. J. and Mah, C. J. (1973). Passive avoidance deficit with septal lesions: Disturbance of response inhibition or response acquisition? *Physiol. Behav.* **11**, 205–213.

Allee, W. C. (1942). Group organization among vertebrates. *Science, N.Y.* **95**, 289–293.

Allikmets, L. H., Vahing, V. A. and Lapin, I. P. (1969). Dissimilar influences of imipramine, benactyzine and promazine on effects of micro-injections of noradrenaline, acetylcholine and serotonin into the amygdala in the cat. *Psychopharmacologia* **15**, 392–403.

Altman, J. (1967). Postnatal growth and differentiation of the mammalian brain, with implications for a morphological theory of memory. In "The Neurosciences", pp. 723–743. (G. C. Quarton, T. Melnechuk and F. O. Schmitt, Eds) Rockefeller University Press, New York.

Amaro, J., Guth, P. S. and Wanderlinder, L. (1966). Inhibition of auditory nerve action potentials by acetylcholine and physostigmine. *Brit. J. Pharmacol. Chemother.* **28**, 207–211.

Anand, B. K. and Brobeck, J. R. (1951). Hypothalamic control of food intake in rats and cats. *Yale J. Biol. Med.* **24**, 123–140.

Andén, N. -E. (1966). On the function of the nigro-neostriatal dopamine pathway. *In* "Mechanism of Release of Biogenic Amines", pp. 357–359. (U.S. Von Euler, S. Rosell and B. Uvnäs, Eds.) Pergamon Press, Oxford.

Andén, N. -E. (1972). Dopamine turnover in the corpus striatum and the limbic system after treatment with neuroleptic and anti-acetylcholine drugs. *J. Pharm. Pharmacol.* **24**, 905–906.

Andén, N. -E., Butcher, S. G., Corrodi, H., Fuxe, K. and Ungerstedt, U. (1970). Receptor activity and turnover of dopamine and noradrenaline after neuroleptics. *Eur. J. Pharmacol.* **11**, 303–314.

Andén, N. -E., Carlsson, A., Dahlstrom, A., Fuxe, K., Hillarp, N. -Å. and Larsson, K. (1964). Demonstration and mapping out of nigro-neostriatal dopamine neurons. *Life Sci.* **3**, 523–530.

Andén, N. -E., Dahlstrom, K., Fuxe, K., Larsson K., Olsen, L. and Ungerstedt, U. (1966). A quantitative study on the nigro-neostriatal dopamine neurone system in the rat. *Acta Physiol. Scand.* **67**, 306–312.

Andersson, B. (1953). The effect of injections of hyperonic NaCl-solutions into different parts of the hypothalamus of goats. *Acta Physiol.aSand.* **28**, 189–201.

Andersson, B. and Jewell, P. A. (1956). The distribtton oι carontid and vertebral blood in the brain and spinal cord of the goat. *Qurt.. J. Exp. Physiol.* **41**, 462–474.

Angelucci, L. (1956). Experiments with perfused frog's spinal cord. *Brit. J. Pharmacol. Chemother.* **11**, 161–170.

Aprison, M. H. and Nathan, P. (1957). Acetylcholine concentrations in the brain of rabbits exhibiting forced turning movements. *Amer. J. Physiol.* **189**, 389–394.

Aprison, M. H., Nathan, P. and Himwich, H. E. (1954a). A study of the relationship between asymmetric acetylcholinesterase activities in rabbit brain and three behavioural patterns. *Science*, N.Y. **119**, 158–159.

Aprison, M. H., Nathan, P. and Himwich, H. E. (1954b). Brain acetylcholinesterase activities in rabbits exhibiting three behavioural patterns following the intracarotid injection of di-isopropyl-fluorophosphate. *Amer. J. Physiol.* **177**, 175–178.

Aprison, M. H., Nathan, P. and Himwich, H. E. (1956). Cholinergic mechanism of brain involved in compulsive circling. *Amer. J. Physiol.* **184**, 244–252.

Aquilonius, S. -M., Lundholm, B. and Winbladh, B. (1972). Effects of some anticholinergic drugs on cortical acetylcholine release and motor activity in rats. *Eur. J. Pharmacol.* **20**, 224–230.

Araki, T., Ito, M., Kostyuk, P. G., Oscarsson, O. and Oshima, T. (1965). The effects of alkaline cations on the responses of cat spinal motoneurones, and their removal from the cells. *Proc. Roy. Soc. B.* **162**, 319–322.

Arbuthnott, G. W. and Crow, T. J. (1971). Relation of contraversive turning to unilateral release of dopamine from the nigro-striatal pathway in rats. *Exp. Neurol.* **30**, 484–491.

Arduini, A. and Arduini, M. G. (1954). Effect of drugs and metabolic alterations on brain stem arousal mechanism. *J. Pharmacol. Exp. Therapeut.* **110**, 76–85.

Arduini, A. and Machne, X. (1949). Sul meccanismo e sul significato dell'azione convulsivante dell'acetilcolina. *Arch. Fisiol.* **48**, 152–167.

Armitage, A. K. and Hall, G. H. (1967). Effects of nicotine on the systemic blood pressure when injected into the cerebral ventricles of cats. *Int. J. Neuropharmacol.* **6**, 143–149.

Armitage, A. K., Hall, G. H. and Sellers, C. M. (1969). Effects of nicotine on electrocortical activity and acetylcholine release from the cat cerebral cortex. *Brit. J. Pharmacol. Chemother.* **35**, 152–160.

Arnfred, T. and Randrup, A. (1968). Cholinergic mechanism in brain inhibiting amphetamine-induced stereotyped behaviour. *Acta Pharmacol. Toxicol.* **26**, 384–394.

Austin, L. and Phillis, J. W. (1965). The distribution of cerebellar cholinesterases in several species. *J. Neurochem.* **12**, 709–717.

Avery, D. D. (1970). Hyperthermia induced by direct injections of carbachol in the anterior hypothalamus. *Neuropharmacology* **9**, 175–178.

Avery, D. D. (1971). Intrahypothalamic adrenergic and cholinergic injection effects on temperature and ingestive behaviour in the rat. *Neuropharmacology* **10**, 753–763.

Baker, W. W., Connor, J. D., Rossi, G. V. and Lalley, P. M. (1967a). Production of tremor by intracaudate cholinergic agents and its suppression by locally administered catecholamines. *Progr. Neuro-Genetics, Vol. 1, Excerpta Medica Int. Congr. Series No.* 175, Amsterdam, pp. 390–403.

Baker, W. W. and Benedict, F. (1967b). Local electrographic responses to intrahippocampal *d*-tubocurarine and related neuromuscular blocking agents. *Proc. Soc. Exp. Biol. Med.* **124**, 607–611.

Baker, W. W. and Benedict, F. (1968a). Analysis of local discharges induced by intrahippocampal micro-injections of carbachol or diisopropyl fluorophosphate (DFP). *Int. J. Neuropharmacol.* **7**, 135–147.

Baker, W. W. and Benedict, F. (1968b). Differential responses of hippocampal repetitive discharges to scopolamine and pentobarbital. *Exp. Neurol.* **21**, 187–200.

Baker, W. W. and Benedict, F. (1970). Influence of increased local cholinergic activity on discharge patterns of hippocampal foci. *EEG Clin. Neurophysiol.* **28**, 499–509.

Baker, W. W., Kratky, M. and Benedict, F. (1965). Electrographic responses to intrahippocampal injections of convulsant drugs. *Exp. Neurol.* **12**, 136–145.

Balazs, R. (1970). Carbohydrate metabolism. *In* "Handbook of Neurochemistry" (A. Lajtha, Ed.) Vol. 3, pp. 1–36, Plenum Press, New York.

Bandler, R. J. (1969). Facilitation of aggressive behaviour in the rat by direct cholinergic stimulation of the hypothalamus. *Nature (Lond.)* **224**, 1035–1036.

Bandler, R. J. (1970). Cholinergic synapses in the lateral hypothalamus for the control of predatory aggression in the rat. *Brain Res.* **20**, 409–424.

Bandler, R. J. (1971a). Direct chemical stimulation of the thalamus: Effects on aggressive behaviour in the rat. *Brain Res.* **26**, 81–93.

Bandler, R. J. (1971b). Chemical stimulation of the rat midbrain and aggressive behaviour. *Nature (Lond.)* **229**, 222–223.

Bandler, R. J., Chi, C. C. and Flynn, J. P. (1972). Biting attack elicited by stimulation of the ventral midbrain tegmentum of cats. *Science, N.Y.* **177**, 364–366.

Barbeau, A. (1962). The pathogenesis of Parkinson's disease; a new hypothesis. *Can. Med. Assn. J.* **87**, 802–807.

Bargmann, W. (1949a). Über die Neurosekretorische Verknupfung von Hypothalamus und Neurohypophyse. *Z. Zellforsch. Abt. Histochem.* **34**, 610–634.

Bargmann, W. (1949b). Über die Neurosekretorische Verknupfung von Hypothalamus und Hypophyse. *Klin. Wschr.* **27**, 617–622.

Barker, J. L., Crayton, J. W. and Nicoll, R. A. (1971a). Supraoptic neurosecretory cells: Autonomic modulation. *Science, N.Y.* **171**, 206–207.

Barker, J. L., Crayton, J. W. and Nicoll, R. A. (1971b). Supraoptic neurosecretory cells: Adrenergic and cholinergic sensitivity. *Science, N.Y.* **171**, 208–210.

Barker, L. A., Amaro, J. and Guth, P. S. (1967). Release of acetylcholine from isolated synaptic vesicles—I. Methods for determining the amount released. *Biochem. Pharmacol.* **16**, 2181–2187.

Bartlett, J. R., Doty, R. W., Pecci-Saavedra, J. and Wilson, P. D. (1973). Mesencephalic control of lateral geniculate nucleus in primates. III. Modification with state of alertness. *Exp. Brain Res.* **18**, 214–224.

Bartolini, A., Bartolini, R. and Pepeu, G. (1970). The effect of oxotremorine on the acetylcholine content of different parts of cat brain. *J. Pharm. Pharmacol.* **22**, 59–60.

Bartolini, A. and Pepeu, G. (1967). Investigations into the acetylcholine output from the cerebral cortex of the cat in the presence of hyoscine. *Brit. J. Pharmacol. Chemother.* **31**, 66–73.

Bartolini, A. and Pepeu, G. (1970). Effect of adrenergic blockers on spontaneous and stimulated acetylcholine output from the cerebral cortex of the cat. *Pharm. Res. Commun.* **2**, 23–29.

Bartolini, A., Weisenthal, L. M. and Domino, E. F. (1972). Effect of photic stimulation on acetycholine release from cat cerebral cortex. *Neuropharmacology* **11**, 113–122.

Batini, C., Moruzzi, G., Palestini, M., Rossi, G. F. and Zanchetti, A. (1958). Persistent patterns of wakefulness in the pretrigeminal midpontine preparation. *Science, N.Y.* **128**, 30–32.

Batini, C., Magni, F., Palestini, M., Rossi, G. F. and Zanchetti, A. (1959a). Neural mechanisms underlying the enduring EEG and behavioral activation in the midpontine pretrigeminal cat. *Archs. Ital. Biol.* **97**, 13–25.

Batini, C., Palestini, M., Rossi, G. F. and Zanchetti, A. (1959b). EEG activation patterns in the midpontine pretrigeminal cat following sensory deafferentation. *Archs. Ital. Biol.* **97**, 26–32.

Baxter, B. L. (1966). Chemical and electrical stimulation of hypothalamic sites mediating "emotional" behavior. *Pharmacologist* **8**, 205.

Beani, L., Bianchi, C., Santinoceto, L. and Marchetti, P. (1968). The cerebral acetylcholine release in conscious rabbits with semi-permanently implanted epidural cups. *Int. J. Neuropharmacol.* **7**, 469–481.

Beckman, A. L. and Carlisle, H. J. (1969). Effects of intrahypothalamic infusion of acetylcholine on behavioral and physiological thermoregulation in the cat. *Nature (Lond.)* **221**, 561–562.

Beleslin, D., Carmichael, A. E. and Feldberg, W. (1964). The origin of acetylcholine appearing in the effluent of perfused cerebral ventricles of the cat. *J. Physiol. (Lond.)* **173**, 368–376.

Beleslin, D. and Myers, R. D. (1970). The release of acetylcholine and 5-hydroxytryptamine from the mesencephalon of the unanaesthetized rhesus monkey. *Brain Res.* **23**, 437–442.

Beleslin, D. and Polak, R. L. (1965). Depression by morphine and chloralose of acetylcholine release from the cat's brain. *J. Physiol. (Lond.)* **177**, 411–419.

Beleslin, D., Polak, R. L. and Sproull, D. H. (1965). The effect of leptazol and strychnine on the acetylcholine release from the cat brain. *J. Physiol. (Lond.)* **181**, 308–316.

Belluzzi, J. D. (1972). Long-lasting effects of cholinergic stimulation of the amygdaloid complex in the rat. *J. Comp. Physiol. Psychol.* **80**, 269–282.

Belluzzi, J. D. and Grossman, S. P. (1969). Avoidance learning: Long-lasting deficits after temporal lobe seizure. *Science, N.Y.* **166**, 1435–1437.

Bennett, E. L., Diamond, M. C., Krech, D. and Rosenzweig, M. R. (1964). Chemical and anatomical plasticity of the brain. *Science, N.Y.* **146**, 610–619.

Bennett, E. L. and Rosenzweig, M. R. (1971). Chemical alterations produced in brain by environment and training. *In* "Handbook of Neurochemistry", Vol. 6, pp. 173–201 (A. Lajtha, Ed.). Plenum Press, New York.

Bennett, T. L. (1973). The effects of centrally blocking hippocampal theta activity on learning and retention. *Behav. Biol.* **9**, 541–552.

Bernheimer, H., Birkmayer, W. und Hornykiewics, O. (1963). Zur Biochemie des Parkinson-Syndroms des Menschen. *Klin. Wschr.* **41**, 465–469.

Bertels–Meeuws, M. M. and Polak, R. L. (1968). Influence of antimuscarinic substances on *in vitro* synthesis of acetylcholine by rat cerebral cortex. *Brit. J. Pharmacol. Chemother.* **33**, 368–380.

Besch, N. F. and Van Dyne, G. C. (1969). Effects of locus and size of septal lesion on consummatory behavior in the rat. *Physiol. Behav.* **4**, 953–958.

Besmedt, J. E. (1962). Auditory-evoked potentials from cochlea to cortex as influenced by activation of the efferent olivo-cochlear bundle. *J. Acoust. Sci.* **34**, 1478–1496.

Bexton, W. H., Heron, W. and Scott, T. H. (1954). Effects of decreased variation in the sensory environment. *Can. J. Psychol.* **8**, 70–76.

Bhattacharya, B. K. and Feldberg, W. (1957). Experiments on perfusion of the ventricular system of the brain in the cat anaesthetized with chloralose. *J. Physiol. (Lond.)* **140**, 5P.

Bhattacharya, B. K. and Feldberg, W. (1958a). Perfusion of cerebral ventricles: Effects of drugs on outflow from the cisterna and the aqueduct. *Brit. J. Pharmacol. Chemother.* **13**, 156–162.

Bhattacharya, B. K. and Feldberg, W. (1958b). Perfusion of cerebral ventricles: Assay of pharmacologically active substances in the effluent from the cisterna and the aqueduct. *Brit. J. Pharmacol. Chemother.* **13**, 163–174.

Bingham, W. E. and Griffiths, W. J. (1952). The effect of different environments during infancy on adult behavior in the rat. *J. Comp. Physiol. Psychol.* **45**, 307–312.

Birks, R. I. (1963). The role of sodium ions in the metabolism of acetycholine. In *Symp. on Function of Acetylcholine as a Synaptic Transmitter*, British Columbia, *Can. J. Biochem. Physiol.* **41**, 2573–2597.

Birks, R. I. and MacIntosh, F. C. (1957). Acetylcholine metabolism at nerve-endings. *Brit. Med. Bull.* **13**, 157–161.

Biscoe, T. J. and Straughan, D. W. (1966). Micro-electrophoretic studies of neurones in the cat hippocampus. *J. Physiol. (Lond.)* **183**, 341–359.

Bisset, G. W. (1968). The milk-ejection reflex and the actions of oxytocin, vasopressin and synthetic analogues on the mammary gland. I. Lactation and the milk-ejection reflex. In "Handbook of Experimental Pharmacology", Vol. XXIII, pp. 475–544. Springer-Verlag, Berlin.

Bisset, G. W. and Lee, J. (1958). Antidiuretic activity in the blood after stimulation of the neurohypophysis in man. *Lancet* **2**, 715–719.

Bisset, G. W. and Walker, J. M. (1957). The effects of nicotine, hexamethonium and ethanol on the secretion of the antidiuretic and oxytocic hormones of the rat. *Brit. J. Pharmacol. Chemother.* **12**, 461–467.

Bjegović, M., Geber, J. and Randić, M. (1969). Effect of tetrodotoxin on the spontaneous release of acetylcholine from the cerebral cortex. *Iugoslav. Physiol. Pharmacol. Acta* **5**, 345–348.

Bjegović, M. and Randić, M. (1971). Effect of lithium ions on the release of acetylcholine from the cerebral cortex. *Nature (Lond.)* **230**, 587–588.

Blass, E. M. and Hanson, D. G. (1970). Primary hyperdipsia in the rat following septal lesions. *J. Comp. Physiol. Psychol.* **70**, 87–93.

Blažević, A., Hadzović, S. and Stern, P. (1965). An experimental contribution to the role of globus pallidus for the occurrence of rest tremor. *Iugoslav, Physiol. Pharmacol. Acta* **1**, 63–68.

Blažević, A., Hamamdžić, M., Magazinović, V. and Stern, P. (1967). The function of motor cells of the anterior horn in the production of rest tremor. *Int. J. Neuropharmacol.* **6**, 119–123.

Bligh, J. (1966). Effects on temperature of monoamines injected into the lateral ventricles of sheep. *J. Physiol. (Lond.)* **185**, 86P.

Boakes, R. J., Bradley, P. B. and Candy, J. M. (1971). Abolition of the responses of brain-stem neurones to iontophoretically applied *d*-amphetamine by reserpine. *Nature (Lond.)* **229**, 496–498.

Bobbin, R. P. and Konishi, T. (1971). Acetylcholine mimics crossed olivocochlear bundle stimulation. *Nature (Lond.)* **231**, NB 222–223.

Booth, D. A. (1968). Mechanism of action of norepinephrine in eliciting an eating response on injection into the rat hypothalamus. *J. Pharmacol. Exp. Therapeut.* **160**, 336–348.

Bordeleau, J. (1961). Système extra-pyramidal et neuroleptiques. Editions Psychiatriques, Montreal.

Borison, H. L. (1961). Respiratory depressant effect of HC-3. *Fed. Proc.* **20**, 594–599.

Bošković, B., Hadžović, S., Krnjević, H. and Stern, P. (1964). Site of production of tremorine effects. *Arch. Int. Pharmacodyn.* **149**, 521–526.

Bourdois, P. S., Mitchell, J. F. and Szerb, J. C. (1971) Effect of atropine on acetylcholine release from cerebral cortical slices stimulated at different frequencies. *Brit. J. Pharmacol. Chemother.* **42**, 640–641P.

Bovet, D. and Longo, V. G. (1956). Pharmacologie de la substance reticulaire. *Abstr. XX Int. Physiol. Congr.* Vol. I. p. 306.

Bowers, M. B. (1967). Factors influencing maintenance and release of acetylcholine in rat cortical brain slices. *Int. J. Neuropharmacol.* **6**, 399–403.

Bradford, H. F. (1968). Carbohydrate and energy metabolism. In "Applied Neurochemistry", pp. 222–250. (A. N. Davison and J. Dobbing, Eds) Blackwell, Oxford.

Bradley, P. B. (1968). The effects of atropine and related drugs on the EEG and behavior. *Progr. Brain Res.* **28**, 3–13.

Bradley, P. B., Cerquiglini, S. and Elkes, J. (1953). Some effects of diisopropylfluoro-phosphate on the electrical activity of the brain in the cat. *J. Physiol. (Lond.)* **121**, 51–52P.

Bradley, P. B., Dhawan, B. N. and Wolstencroft, J. H. (1966). Pharmacological properties of cholinoceptive neurones in the medulla and pons of the cat. *J. Physiol. (Lond.)* **183**, 658–674.

Bradley, P. B. and Elkes, J. (1953). The effect of amphetamine and D-lysergic acid diethylamide (LSD-25) on the electrical activity of the brain of the conscious cat. *J. Physiol. (Lond.)* **120**, 13P.

Bradley, P. B. and Elkes, J. (1957). The effects of some drugs on the electrical activity of the brain. *Brain* **80**, 77–117.

Bradley, P. B. and Nicholson, A. N. (1962). The effect of some drugs on hippocampal arousal. *EEG Clin. Neurophysiol.* **14**, 824–834.

Bradley, P. B. and Wolstencroft, J. H. (1962). Excitation and inhibition of brain-stem neurons by nor-adrenaline and acetylcholine. *Nature (Lond.)* **196**, 840.

Bradley, P. B. and Wolstencroft, J. H. (1965). Actions of drugs on single neurones in the brainstem. *Brit. Med. Bull.* **21**, 15–18.

Brady, J. V. (1961). Motivational-emotional factors and intracranial self-stimulation. *In* "Electrical Stimulation of the Brain", pp. 413–430. (D. Sheer, Ed.) University of Texas Press, Austin.

Brady, J. V., Boren, J. J., Conrad, D. G. and Sidman, M. (1957). The effect of food and water deprivation upon intracranial self-stimulation. *J. Comp. Physiol. Psychol.* **50**, 134–137.

Brady, J. V. and Nauta, W. J. H. (1953). Subcortical mechanisms in emotional behavior: Affective changes following septal forebrain lesions in the albino rat. *J. Comp. Physiol. Psychol.* **46**, 339–346.

Braganca, B. M. and Quastel, J. H. (1952). Action of snake venom on acetylcholine synthesis in brain. *Nature (Lond.)* **169**, 695–697.

Brazeau, P. (1971). *In* "The Pharmacological Basis of Therapeutics", pp. 874–885. (L. S. Goodman and A. Gilman, Eds) 4th Edn, Macmillan, London.

Breen, R. A. and McGaugh, J. L. (1961). Facilitation of maze learning with post trial injections of picrotoxin. *J. Comp. Physiol. Psychol.* **54**, 498–501.

Bremer, F. (1937). L'activité cérébrale au cours du sommeil et de la narcose. Contribution a l'étude du mécanisme du sommeil. *Bull. Acad. Roy. Med. Belgique* **2**, 68–86.

Bremer, F. and Stoupel, N. (1959). Etude pharmacologique de la facilitation des réponses corticales dans l'éveil réticulaire. *Arch. Int. Pharmacodyn.* **122**, 234–248.

Brezenoff, H. E. (1972). Cardiovascular responses to intrahypothalamic injections of carbachol and certain cholinesterase inhibitors. *Neuropharmacology* **11**, 637–644.

Brezenoff, H. E. and Jenden, D. J. (1969). Modification of arterial blood pressure in rats following microinjection of drugs into the posterior hypothalamus. *Int. J. Neuropharmacol.* **8**, 593–600.

Brezenoff, H. E. and Jenden, D. J. (1970). Changes in arterial blood pressure after microinjections of carbachol into the medulla and IVth ventricle of the rat brain. *Neuropharmacology* **9**, 341–348.

Brezenoff, H. E. and Wirecki, T. S. (1970). The pharmacological specificity of muscarinic receptors in the posterior hypothalamus of the rat. *Life Sci.* **9**, 99–109.

Brodie, B. B. and Shore, P. A. (1957). A concept for the role of serotonin and nor-epinephrine as chemical mediators in the brain. *Ann. N.Y. Acad. Sci.* **66**, 631–642.

Brody, J. F., DeFeudis, P. A. and DeFeudis, F. V. (1969). Effects of micro-injections of L-glutamate into the hypothalamus on attack and flight behaviours in cats. *Nature (Lond.)* **224**, 1330.

Brooks, C. McC., Ishikawa, T., Koizumi, K. and Lu, H. H. (1966). Activity of neurones in the paraventricular nucleus of the hypothalamus and its control. *J. Physiol.* (*Lond.*) **182**, 217–231.

Brooks, V. B., Ransmeier, R. E. and Gerard, R. W. (1949). Action of anticholinesterases, drugs and intermediates on respiration and electrical activity of the isolated frog brain. *Amer. J. Physiol.* **157**, 299–316.

Brown, C. P. (1971). Cholinergic activity in rats following enriched stimulation and training. *J. Comp. Physiol. Psychol.* **75**, 408–416.

Browning, E. T. and Schulman, M. P. (1968). [$^{14}$C] Acetylcholine synthesis by cortex slices of rat brain. *J. Neurochem.* **15**, 1391–1405.

Brownlee, W. C. and Mitchell, J. F. (1968). The pharmacology of cortical repetitive after discharges. *Brit. J. Pharmacol. Chemother.* **33**, 217–218P.

Brücke, F., Gogolák, G. and Stumpf, Ch. (1963). Mikroelektrodenuntersuchung der Reizantwort und der Zelltatigkeit im Hippocampus bei Septumreizung. *Pflüg. Arch.* **276**, 456–470.

Bülbring, E. and Burn, J. H. (1941). Observations bearing on synaptic transmission by acetylcholine in the spinal cord. *J. Physiol.* (*Lond.*) **100**, 337–368.

Burdick, C. J. and Strittmatter, C. F. (1965). Appearance of biochemical components related to acetylcholine metabolism during the embryonic development of chick brain. *Archs. Biochem. Biophys.* **109**, 293–301.

Bureš, J. B., Bohdanecký, Z. and Weiss, T. (1962). Physostigmine-induced hippocampal theta activity and learning in rats. *Psychopharmacologia* **3**, 254–263.

Burgen, A. S. V. and Chipman, L. M. (1951). Cholinesterase and succinic dehydrogenase in the central nervous system of the dog. *J. Physiol.* (*Lond.*) **114**, 296–305.

Burks, C. D. and Fisher, A. E. (1970). Anticholinergic blockade of schedule-induced polydipsia. *Physiol. Behav.* **5**, 635–640.

Burn, G. P. and Grewal, R. S. (1951). The antidiuretic response to and excretion of pituitary (posterior lobe) extract in man, with reference to the action of nicotine. *Brit. J. Pharmacol. Chemother.* **6**, 471–482.

Burn, J. H., Truelove, L. H. and Burn, I. (1945). Antidiuretic action of nicotine and of smoking. *Brit. Med. J.* **1**, 403–406.

Burns, B. D. (1954). The production of afterbursts in isolated unanaesthetized cerebral cortex. *J. Physiol.* (*Lond.*) **125**, 427–446.

Burns, B. D. (1958). "The Mammalian Cerebral Cortex". Arnold, London.

Burns, N. M. and Kimura, D. (1963). Isolation and sensory deprivation. *In* "Unusual Environments and Human Behavior", pp. 167–192. (N. M. Burns, R. M. Chambers and E. Hendler, Eds), Free Press of Glencoe, Collier-Macmillan, London.

Campbell, L. B., Hanin, I. and Jenden, D. J. (1970). Gas chromatographic evaluation of the effects of some muscarinic and anti-muscarinic drugs on acetylcholine levels in rat brain. *Biochem. Pharmacol.* **19**, 2053–2059.

Carlton, P. L. (1963). Cholinergic mechanisms in the control of behaviour by the brain. *Psychol. Rev.* **70**, 19–39.

Carlton, P. L. (1969). Brain acetylcholine and inhibition. *In* "Reinforcement: Current Research and Theories", pp. 286–327. (J. Tapp. Ed.) Academic Press, New York and London.

Carmichael, E. A., Feldberg, W. and Fleischauer, K. (1962). The site of origin of the tremor produced by tubocurarine acting from the cerebral ventricles. *J. Physiol.* (*Lond.*) **172**, 539–554.

Celesia, G. G. and Jasper, H. H. (1966). Acetylcholine released from the cerebral cortex in relation to state of activation. *Neurology* (*Minneap.*) **16**, 1053–1063.

Chakrin, L. W., Marchbanks, R. M., Mitchell, J. F. and Whittaker, V. P. (1972). The origin of the acetylcholine released from the surface of the cortex. *J. Neurochem.* **19**, 2727–2736.

Chalmers, R. K. and Erickson, C. K. (1964). Central cholinergic blockade of the conditioned avoidance response in rats. *Psychopharmacologia* **6**, 31–41.

Chalmers, R. K. and Yim, G. K. W. (1963). Spinal action of tremorine in the dog. *Arch. Int. Pharmacodyn.* **145**, 322–333.

Chalmers, T. M. and Lewis, A. A. G. (1951). Stimulation of the supraoptico-hypophysial system in man. *Clin. Sci.* **10**, 127–135.

Chang, H. -C., Chia, K. -F., Hsu, C. -H. and Lim, R. K. S. (1937a). Reflex secretion of the posterior pituitary elicited through the vagus. *J. Physiol. (Lond.)* **90**, 87–89P.

Chang, H. -C., Chia, K. -F., Hsu, C. -H. and Lim, R. K. S. (1937b). Humoral transmission of nerve impulses at central synapses. I. Sinus and vagus afferent nerves. *Chin. J. Physiol.* **12**, 1–36.

Chang, H. -C., Chia, K. -F., Hsu, C. -H. and Lim, R. K. S. (1937c). A vagus-postpituitary reflex. *Chin. J. Physiol.* **12**, 309–326.

Chang, H. -C., Chia, K. -F., Hsu, C. -H. and Lim, R. K. S. (1938a). Humoral transmission of nerve impulses at central synapses. II. Central vagus transmission after hypophysectomy in the dog. *Chin. J. Physiol.* **13**, 13–32.

Chang, H. -C., Lim, R. K. S., Lu, T. -M., Wang, C. -C. and Wang, K. -J. (1938b). A vagus-post-pituitary reflex. III. Oxytocic component. *Chin. J. Physiol.* **13**, 269–284.

Chapman, J. B. and McCance, I. (1967). Acetylcholine-sensitive cells in the intracerebellar nuclei of the cat. *Brain Res.* **5**, 535–538.

Chatfield, P. O. and Dempsey, E. W. (1942). Some effects of prostigmine and acetylcholine on cortical potentials. *Amer. J. Physiol.* **135**, 633–640.

Cheney, D. L., Gubler, C. J. and Jaussi, A. W. (1969). Production of acetylcholine in rat brain following thiamine deprivation and treatment with thiamine antagonists. *J. Neurochem.* **16**, 1283–1291.

Chiou, C. Y., Long, J. P., Potrepka, R. and Spratt, J. L. (1970). The ability of various nicotinic agents to release acetylcholine from synaptic vesicles. *Arch. Int. Pharmacodyn.* **187**, 88–96.

Cho, A. K., Haslett, W. L. and Jenden, D. J. (1961). The identification of an active metabolite of tremorine. *Biochem. Biophys. Res. Commun.* **5**, 276–279.

Cho, A. K., Haslett, W. L. and Jenden, D. J. (1962). The peripheral actions of oxotremorine, a metabolite of tremorine. *J. Pharmacol. Exp. Therapeut.* **138**, 249–257.

Chorova, S. L. and Schiller, P. H. (1965). Short-term retrograde amnesia in rats. *J. Comp. Physiol. Psychol.* **59**, 73–78.

Christian, J. J. (1963). Endocrine adaptive mechanisms and the physiologic regulation of population growth. *In* "Physiological Mammalogy", Vol. 1, pp. 189–353, Academic Press, New York and London.

Chronister, R. B., Bernstein, J. J., Zornetzer, S. F. and White, L. E. Jr. (1973). Synaptic boutons in the hippocampus: Changes are produced by age and experience. *Experientia*, **29**, 588–589.

Churchill, J. A., Schuknecht, H. F. and Doran, R. (1956). Acetylcholinesterase activity in the cochlea. *Laryngoscope (St. Louis)* **66**, 1–15.

Collier, B. (1970). Biosynthesis of acetylcholine *in vitro* and *in vivo*. *In* "Drugs and Cholinergic Mechanisms in the CNS", pp. 163–176. (B. Holmstedt, J. Schuberth, B. Sorbo, and A. Sundwall, Eds) Försvarets Forskningsanstalt, Stockholm.

Collier, B. and Mitchell, J. F. (1966). The central release of acetylcholine during stimulation of the visual pathway. *J. Physiol. (Lond.)* **184**, 239–254.

Collier, B. and Mitchell, J. F. (1967). The central release of acetylcholine during consciousness and after brain lesions. *J. Physiol. (Lond.)* **188**, 83–98.

Collier, B. and Murray-Brown, N. (1968). Validity of a method measuring transmitter release from the central nervous system. *Nature (Lond.)* **218**, 434–435.

Connor, J. D., Rossi, G. V. and Baker, W. W. (1966a). Characteristics of tremor in cats following carbachol injections into the caudate nucleus. *Exp. Neurol.* **14**, 371–382.

Connor, J. D., Rossi, G. V. and Baker, W. W. (1966b). Analysis of the tremor induced by injection of cholinergic agents into the caudate nucleus. *Int. J. Neuropharmacol.* **5**, 207–216.

Connor, J. D., Rossi, G. V. and Baker, W. W. (1967). Antagonism of intracaudate carbachol tremor by local injections of catecholamines. *J. Pharmacol. Exp. Therapeut.* **155**, 545–551.

Consolo, S. and Valzelli, L. (1970). Brain choline acetylase and monoamine oxidase activity in normal and aggressive mice. *Eur. J. Pharmacol.* **13**, 129–130.

Cools, A. R. and Van Rossum, M. J. (1970). Caudal dopamine and stereotype behaviour of cats. *Arch. Int. Pharmacodyn.* **187**, 163–173.

Cooper, K. E. (1966). Temperature regulation and the hypothalamus. *Brit. Med. Bull.* **2**, 238–242.

Cooper, K. E., Cranston, W. I. and Honour, A. J. (1965). Effects of intraventricular and intrahypothalamic injections of noradrenaline and 5-HT on body temperature in conscious rabbits. *J. Physiol. (Lond.)* **181**, 852–864.

Cordeau, J. P. and Mancia, M. (1958). Effect of unilateral chronic lesions of the midbrain on the electrocortical activity of the cat. *Archs. Ital. Biol.* **96**, 374–399.

Costall, B. and Naylor, R. J. (1973). Is there a relationship between the involvement of extrapyramidal and mesolimbic brain areas with the cataleptic action of neuroleptic agents and their clinical antipsychotic effect? *Psychopharmacologia* **32**, 161–170.

Costall, B., Naylor, R. J. and Olley, J. E. (1972). Catalepsy and circling behaviour after intracerebral injections of neuroleptic, cholinergic and anticholinergic agents into the caudate-putamen, globus pallidus and substantia nigra of rat brain. *Neuropharmacolology* **11**, 645–663.

Costall, B. and Olley, J. E. (1971a). Cholinergic and neuroleptic induced catalepsy: Modifications by lesions in the caudate-putamen. *Neuropharmacology* **10**, 297–306.

Costall, B. and Olley, J. E. (1971b). Cholinergic and neuroleptic induced catalepsy: Modification by lesions in the globus pallidus and substantia nigra. *Neuropharmacology* **10**, 581–594.

Cottle, M. K. W. and Silver, A. (1970). Histochemical demonstration of acetylcholinesterase in the hypothalamus of the female guinea-pig. *Z. Zellforsch.* **103**, 570–588.

Coury, J. N. (1967). Neural correlates of food and water intake in the rat. *Science, N.Y.* **156**, 1763–1765.

Cox, B. and Potkonjak, D. (1969). An investigation of tremorgenic effects of oxotremorine and tremorine after stereotaxic injection into rat brain. *Int. J. Neuropharmacol.* **8**, 291–297.

Crawford, J. M., Curtis, D. R., Voorhoeve, P. E. and Wilson, V. J. (1966). Acetylcholine sensitivity of cerebellar neurones in the cat. *J. Physiol. (Lond.)* **185**, 139–165.

Crawshaw, L. I. (1973). Effect of intracranial acetylcholine injection on thermoregulatory responses in the rat. *J. Comp. Physiol. Psychol.* **83**, 32–35.

Cross, B. A. and Green, J. D. (1959). Activity of single neurons in the hypothalamus: Effect of osmotic and other stimuli. *J. Physiol. (Lond.)* **148**, 554–569.

Crossland, J. (1953). The significance of brain acetylcholine. *J. Ment. Sci.* **99**, 247–251.

Crossland, J. and Merrick, A. J. (1954). The effect of anaesthesia on the acetylcholine content of brain. *J. Physiol. (Lond.)* **125**, 56–66.

Curtis, D. R. and Crawford, J. M. (1969). Central synaptic transmission—Micro-electrophoretic studies. *Ann. Rev. Pharmacol.* **9,** 209–240.

Curtis, D. R. and Eccles, R. M. (1958a). The excitation of Renshaw cells by pharmacological agents applied electrophoretically. *J. Physiol. (Lond.)* **141,** 435–445.

Curtis, D. R. and Eccles, R. M. (1958b). The effect of diffusional barriers upon the pharmacology of cells within the central nervous system. *J. Physiol. (Lond.)* **141,** 446–463.

Curtis, D. R., Eccles, J. C. and Eccles, R. M. (1957). Pharmacological studies on spinal reflexes. *J. Physiol. (Lond.)* **136,** 420–434.

Curtis, D. R. and Phillis, J. W. (1960). The action of procaine and atropine on spinal neurones. *J. Physiol. (Lond.)* **153,** 17–34.

Curtis, D. R., Phillis, J. W. and Watkins, J. C. (1961). Cholinergic and non-cholinergic transmission in the mammalian spinal cord. *J. Physiol. (Lond.)* **158,** 296–323.

Daigneault, E. A. and Brown, R. D. (1966). Acetylcholine suppression of the $N_1$ component of round window recorded cochlear potentials. *Arch. Int. Pharmacodyn.* **162,** 20–29.

David, J. P., Murayama, S., Machne, X. and Unna, K. R. (1963). Evidence supporting cholinergic transmission at the lateral geniculate body of the cat. *Int. J. Neuropharmacol.* **2,** 113–125.

DeBoor, W. (1956). "Pharmakopsychologie und Psychopathologie". Springer, Berlin.

Decsi, L. and Várszegi, M. K. (1969). Fear and escape reaction evoked by the intra-hypothalamic injection of *d*-tubocurarine in unrestrained cats. *Acta Physiol. Acad. Sci. Hung.* **36,** 95–104.

DeFeudis, F. V. (1971). Effects of environmental changes on the incorporation of carbon atoms of D-glucose into mouse brain and other tissues. *Life Sci.* **10** (Part II) 1187–1194.

DeFeudis, F. V. (1972). Effects of isolation and aggregation on the incorporation of carbon atoms of D-mannose and D-glucose into mouse brain. *Biol. Psychiat.* **4,** 239–242.

DeFeudis, F. V. (1973). Effects of *d*-amphetamine on the incorporation of carbon atoms of D-mannose into the brains and sera of differentially-housed mice. *Biol. Psychiat.* **7,** 3–9.

DeFeudis, F. V. (1974). Cerebral biochemical and pharmacological changes in differentially-housed mice. *In* "Current Developments in Psychopharmacology" Vol. 1. (W. B. Essman and L. Valzelli, Eds) Spectrum Publications, New York.

Deffenu, G., Bartolini, A. and Pepeu, G. (1970). Effect of amphetamine on cholinergic systems of the cerebral cortex of the cat. *In* "Amphetamines and Related Compounds", pp. 357–368. (E. Costa and S. Garattini, Eds) Raven Press, New York.

Deffenu, G., Bertaccini, G. and Pepeu, G. (1967). Acetylcholine and 5-hydroxytryptamine levels of the lateral geniculate bodies and superior colliculus of cats after visual deafferentation. *Exp. Neurol.* **17,** 203–209.

Deffenu, G., Mantegazzini, P. and Pepeu, G. (1966). Scopolamine-induced changes of brain acetylcholine and EEG pattern in cats with complete pontine transection. *Archs. Ital. Biol.* **104,** 141–151.

del Castillo, J. and Katz, B. (1954). The effect of magnesium on the activity of motor nerve endings. *J. Physiol. (Lond.)* **124,** 553–559.

del Castillo, J. and Katz, B. (1956). Biophysical aspects of neuromuscular transmission. *Progr. Biophys.* **6,** 121–170.

Delgado, J. M. R. (1965). Sequential behavior induced repeatedly by stimulation of the red nucleus in free monkeys. *Science, N.Y.* **148,** 1361–1363.

Delgado, J. M. R. (1966). Intracerebral perfusion in awake monkeys. *Arch. Int. Pharmacodyn.* **161,** 442–462.

Delgado, J. M. R. and Anand, B. K. (1953). Increase of food intake induced by electrical stimulation of the lateral hypothalamus. *Amer. J. Physiol.* **172**, 162–168.

Delgado, J. M. R. and DeFeudis, F. V. (1969). Effects of lithium injections into the amygdala and hippocampus of awake monkeys. *Exp. Neurol.* **25**, 255–267.

Delgado, J. M. R. and Rubinstein, L. (1964). Intracerebral release of neurohumors in unanesthetized monkeys. *Arch. Int. Pharmacodyn.* **150**, 530–546.

Dement, W. (1958). The occurrence of low voltage, fast electroencephalogram patterns during behavioural sleep in the cat. *EEG Clin. Neurophysiol.* **10**, 291–296.

Dempsey, E. W. and Morrison, R. S. (1942). The production of rhythmically recurrent cortical potentials after localized thalamic stimulation. *Amer. J. Physiol.* **135**, 293–300.

Dempsey, E. W. and Morrison, R. S. (1943). The electrical activity of a thalamocortical relay system. *Amer. J. Physiol.* **138**, 283–298.

Denisenko, P. P. (1962). Influence of pharmacological agents upon cholinoreactive and adrenoreactive systems of the reticular formation and other regions of the brain. *In* "Pharmacological Analysis of Central Nervous Action", pp. 199–201. (W. D. M. Paton Ed.) Vol. 8, Macmillan, New York.

De Robertis, E. D. P. (1964). "Histophysiology of Synapses and Neurosecretion". Pergamon Press, Oxford.

Deutsch, J. A. (1966). Substrates of learning and memory. *Dis. of the CNS* **27**, 20–24.

Deutsch, J. A. (1969). The physiological basis of memory. *Ann. Rev. Psychol.* **20**, 85–104.

Deutsch, J. A. (1971). The cholinergic synapse and the site of memory. *Science, N.Y.* **174**, 788–794.

Deutsch, J. A., Hamburg, M. D. and Dahl, H. (1966). Anticholinesterase-induced amnesia and its temporal aspects. *Science, N.Y.* **151**, 221–223.

Deutsch, J. A. and Leibowitz, S. F. (1966). Amnesia or reversal of forgetting by anticholinesterase, depending simply on time of injection. *Science, N.Y.* **153**, 1017–1018.

Deutsch, J. A. and Rocklin, K. W. (1967). Amnesia induced by scopolamine and its temporal variations. *Nature (Lond.)* **216**, 89–90.

DeWeid, D. (1966). Effect of autonomic blocking agents and structurally related substances on the "salt arousal of drinking". *Physiol. Behav.* **1**, 193–197.

Diamond, M. C., Krech, D. and Rosenzweig, M. R. (1964). The effects of an enriched environment on the histology of the rat cerebral cortex. *J. Comp. Neurol.* **123**, 111–120.

Diamond, M. C., Law, F., Rhodes, H., Lindner, B., Rosenzweig, M. R., Krech, D. and Bennett, E. L. (1966). Increases in cortical depth and glia numbers in rats subjected to enriched environment. *J. Comp. Neurol.* **128**, 117–126.

Diezel, P. B. and Taubert, M. (1954). Untersuchungen am Gehirneisen. *Verh. dtsch. Ges. Path.* **38**, 321–326.

Dikshit, B. B. (1934a). Action of acetylcholine on the brain and its occurrence therein. *J. Physiol. (Lond.)* **80**, 409–421.

Dikshit, B. B. (1934b). The production of cardiac irregularities by excitation of the hypothalamic centres. *J. Physiol. (Lond.)* **81**, 382–394.

Dikshit, B. B. (1934c). Action of acetylcholine on the "sleep centre". *J. Physiol. (Lond.)* **83**, 42P.

Dikshit, B. B. (1935). The physiology of sleep. *Lancet* **228**, (I), 570.

Dill, R. E., Nickey, W. M. and Little, M. D. (1968). Dyskinesias in rats following chemical stimulation of the neostriatum. *Texas Rep. Biol. Med.* **26**, 101–106.

Domino, E. F. (1966). Role of cholinergic mechanisms in states of wakefulness and sleep. *In* "Proc. 5th Int. Congr. Coll. Int. Neuropsychopharmacol", pp. 378–379, Washington, D.C., Excerpta Med. Int. Congr. Series, No. 129.

Domino, E. F. (1967). Electroencephalographic and behavioral arousal effect of small doses of nicotine: A neuropsychopharmacological study. *Ann. N.Y. Acad. Sci.* **142**, 216–244.

Domino, E. F. (1968). Role of the central cholinergic system in wakefulness, fast wave sleep and "no-go" behavior. *In* "The Present Status of Psychotropic Drugs", pp. 273–277, Excerpta Med. Int. Congr. Series, No. 180.

Domino, E. F. and Bartolini, A. (1972). Effects of various psychotomimetic agents on the EEG and acetylcholine release from the cerebral cortex of brainstem transected cats. *Neuropharmacology* **11**, 703–713.

Domino, E. F., Dren, A. T. and Yamamoto, K. I. (1967). Pharmacologic evidence for cholinergic mechanisms in neocortical and limbic activating systems. *Progr. Brain Res.* **27**, 337–364.

Domino, E. F. and Hudson, R. D. (1958). Observations on the pharmacological actions of the isomers of atropine. *J. Pharmacol. Exp. Therapeut.* **127**, 305–312.

Domino, E. F. and Olds, M. E. (1968). Cholinergic inhibition of self-stimulation behavior. *J. Pharmacol. Exp. Therapeut.* **164**, 202–211.

Domino, E. F. and Olds, M. E. (1972). Effects of D-amphetamine, scopolamine, chlordiazepoxide and diphenylhydantoin on self-stimulation behavior and brain acetylcholine. *Psychopharmacologia* **23**, 1–16.

Domino, E. F., Yamamoto, K. and Dren, A. T. (1968). Role of cholinergic mechanisms in states of wakefulness and sleep. *Progr. Brain Res.* **28**, 113–133.

Doty, B. A. and Johnston, M. M. (1966). Effects of posttrial eserine administration, age and task difficulty on avoidance conditioning in rats. *Psychonom. Sci.* **6**, 101–102.

Doty, R. W., Wilson, P. D., Bartlett, J. R. and Pecci-Saavedra, J. (1973). Mesencephalic control of lateral geniculate nucleus in primates. I. Electrophysiology. *Exp. Brain Res.* **18**, 189–203.

Dreifuss, J. J. and Kelly, J. S. (1972a). Recurrent inhibition of antidromically identified rat supraoptic neurones. *J. Physiol. (Lond.)* **220**, 87–103.

Dreifuss, J. J. and Kelly, J. S. (1972b). The activity of identified supraoptic neurones and their response to acetylcholine applied by iontophoresis. *J. Physiol. (Lond.)* **220**, 105–118.

Dren, A. T. and Domino, E. F. (1968). Effects of hemicholinium (HC-3) on EEG activation and brain acetylcholine in the dog. *J. Pharmacol. Exp. Therapeut.* **161**, 141–154.

Dubinsky, B. and Goldberg, M. E. (1971). The effect of imipramine and selected drugs on attack elicited by hypothalamic stimulation in the cat. *Neuropharmacology* **10**, 537–545.

Dudar, J. D. and Szerb, J. C. (1969). The effect of topically applied atropine on resting and evoked cortical acetylcholine release. *J. Physiol. (Lond.)* **203**, 741–762.

Duke, H. N. and Pickford, M. (1951). Observations on the action of acetylcholine and adrenaline on the hypothalamus. *J. Physiol. (Lond.)* **114**, 325–332.

Duke, H. N., Pickford, M. and Watt, J. A. (1950). The immediate and delayed effects of diisopropyl fluorophosphate injected into the supraoptic nuclei of dogs. *J. Physiol. (Lond.)* **111**, 81–88.

Duncan, C. P. (1949). The retroactive effect of electroshock on learning. *J. Comp. Physiol. Psychol.* **42**, 32–44.

Dyball, R. E. J. (1971). Oxytocin and ADH secretion in relation to electrical activity in antidromically identified supraoptic and paraventricular units. *J. Physiol. (Lond.)* **214**, 245–256.

Dyball, R. E. J. and Koizumi, K. (1969). Electrical activity in the supraoptic and paraventricular nuclei associated with neurohypophysial hormone release. *J. Physiol. (Lond.)* **201**, 711–722.

Eccles, J. C. (1964). "The Physiology of Synapses". Academic Press, New York and London.

Eccles, J. C. (1969). "The Inhibitory Pathways of the Central Nervous System (The Sherrington Lectures, IX)" 135 pp. Liverpool.

Eccles, J. C., Eccles, R. M. and Fatt, P. (1956). Pharmacological investigations on a central synapse operated by acetylcholine. *J. Physiol. (Lond.)* **131**, 154–169.

Eccles, J. C., Fatt, P. and Koketsu, K. (1954). Cholinergic and inhibitory synapses in a pathway from motor-axon collaterals to motoneurones. *J. Physiol. (Lond.)* **126**, 524–562.

Edery, H. and Levinger, I. M. (1971). Acetylcholine release into the perfused intermeningeal spaces of the cat spinal cord. *Neuropharmacology* **10**, 239–246.

Ehringer, H. and Hornykiewics, O. (1960). Verteilung von Noradrenaline und Dopamin (3-Hydroxytyramin) im Gehirn des Menschen und ihr Verhalten bei Erkrankungen des Extrapyramidalen Systems. *Klin. Wschr.* **38**, 1236–1239.

Elie, R. and Panisset, J. -C. (1970). Effect of angiotensin and atropine on the spontaneous release of acetylcholine from cat cerebral cortex. *Brain Res.* **17**, 297–305.

Elliott, K. A. C., Swank, R. L. and Henderson, N. (1950). Effect of anaesthetics and convulsants on acetylcholine content of brain. *Amer. J. Physiol.* **162**, 469–474.

Elliott, K. A. C. and Wolfe, L. S. (1962). Brain tissue respiration and glycolysis. *In* "Neurochemistry", pp. 177–211. (K. A. C. Elliott, I. H. Page and J. H. Quastel, Eds), 2nd Ed., C. C. Thomas, Springfield, Illinois.

Emerson, G. A. and Tischler, M. (1944). The antiriboflavin effect of isoriboflavin. *Proc. Soc. Exp. Biol. Med.* **55**, 184–185.

Endröczi, E., Hartmann, G. and Lissák, K. (1963). Effect of intracerebrally administered cholinergic and adrenergic drugs on neocortical and archicortical electrical activity. *Acta Physiol. Acad. Sci. Hung.* **24**, 199–210.

Epstein, A. N., Fitzsimons, J. T. and Rolls, B. J. (1970). Drinking induced by injection of angiotensin into the brain of the rat. *J. Physiol. (Lond.)* **210**, 457–474.

Erdmann, W. D. and Teutloff, K. (1963). Atropin-Ersatzstoffe in der Therapie von Alkylphosphat-Vergiftungen an Ratten. *Arzneimittelforsch.* **13**, 381–383.

Erulkar, S. D., Nichols, C. W., Popp, M. B. and Koelle, G. B. (1968). Renshaw elements: Localisation and acetylcholinesterase content. *J. Histochem. Cytochem.* **16**, 128–135.

Essig, C. F., Hampson, J. L. and Himwich, H. E. (1953). Biochemically induced circling behavior. *Confin. Neurol.* **13**, 65–70.

Essig, C. F., Hampson, J. L., McCauley, A. and Himwich, H. E. (1950). An experimental analysis of biochemically induced circling behavior. *J. Neurophysiol.* **13**, 269–275.

Essman, W. B. (1971). Changes in cholinergic activity and avoidance behavior by nicotine in differentially housed mice. *Int. J. Neurosci.* **2**, 199–206.

Essman, W. B. (1972). Contributions of differential housing to brain development: Some implications for sleep behavior. *In* "Sleep and the Maturing Nervous System", pp. 99–107. (C. D. Clemente, D. P. Purpura and F. E. Mayer, Eds) Academic Press, New York and London.

Everett, G. M. (1956). Tremor produced by drugs. *Nature (Lond.)* **177**, 1238.

Everett, G. M. (1961). Tremorine. "Extrapyramidal system and neuroleptica". Editions Psychiatriques, Montreal.

Fahn, S. and Coté, L. J. (1968). Regional distribution of choline acetylase in the brain of the rhesus monkey. *Brain Res.* **7**, 323–325.

Falk, J. L. (1961). Production of polydipsia in normal rats by an intermittent food schedule. *Science, N.Y.* **133**, 195–196.

Feldberg, W. (1945). Present views on the mode of action of acetylcholine in the central nervous system. *Physiol. Rev.* **25**, 596–642.

Feldberg, W. (1950). The role of acetylcholine in the central nervous system. *Brit. Med. Bull.* **6**, 312–321.

Feldberg, W. (1954). Central and sensory transmission. *Pharmacol. Rev.* **6**, 85–93.

Feldberg, W. and Fleischauer, K. (1962). The site of origin of the seizure discharge produced by tubocurarine acting from the cerebral ventricles. *J. Physiol. (Lond.)* **160**, 258–283.

Feldberg, W. and Fleischauer, K. (1963). The hippocampus as the site of origin of the seizure discharge produced by tubocurarine acting from the cerebral ventricles. *J. Physiol. (Lond.)* **168**, 435–442.

Feldberg, W. and Fleischauer, K. (1965). A new experimental approach to the physiology and pharmacology of the brain. *Brit. Med. Bull.* **21**, 36–43.

Feldberg, W. and Malcolm, J. L. (1959). Experiments on the site of action of tubocurarine when applied via the cerebral ventricles. *J. Physiol. (Lond.)* **149**, 58–77.

Feldberg, W. and Myers, R. D. (1964). Effects on temperature of amines injected into the cerebral ventricles. A new concept of temperature regulation. *J. Physiol. (Lond.)* **173**, 226–237.

Feldberg, W. and Myers, R. D. (1965). Changes in temperature produced by microinjections of amines into the anterior hypothalamus of cats. *J. Physiol. (Lond.)* **177**, 239–245.

Feldberg, W. and Sherwood, S. L. (1954). Injections of drugs into the lateral ventricle of the cat. *J. Physiol. (Lond.)* **123**, 148–167.

Feldberg, W. and Vogt, M. (1948). Acetylcholine synthesis in different regions of the central nervous system. *J. Physiol. (Lond.)* **107**, 372–381.

Fex, J. (1962). Auditory activity in centrifugal and centripetal cochlear fibres in cat. *Acta Physiol. Scand.* **55**, Suppl. No. 189.

Fex, J. (1968). Efferent inhibition in the cochlea by the olivo-cochlear bundle. *In* "Ciba Fdn. Symp. Hearing Mechanisms in Vertebrates", pp. 169–186. (A. V. S. de Reuck and J. Knight, Eds) Little, Brown and Co., Boston.

Fibiger, H. C., Lytle, L. D. and Campbell, B. A. (1970). Cholinergic modulation of adrenergic arousal in the developing rat. *J. Comp. Physiol. Psychol.* **72**, 384–389.

Fifková, E. and Maršala, J. (1967). Stereotaxic atlas for the rat brain. *In* "Electrophysiological Methods in Biological Research", pp. 653–695. (J. Bureš, M. Petrán and J. Zachar, Eds) Academic Press, New York and London.

Fisher, A. E. and Coury, J. N. (1962). Cholinergic tracing of a central neural circuit underlying the thirst drive. *Science, N.Y.* **138**, 691–693.

Fisher, A. E. and Coury, J. N. (1964). Chemical tracing of neural pathways mediating the thirst drive. *In* "Thirst", pp. 515–531. (M. J. Wayner, Ed.) Pergamon Press, Oxford.

Fitzsimons, J. T. (1961). Drinking by rats depleted of body fluid without increase in osmotic pressure. *J. Physiol. (Lond.)* **159**, 297–309.

Fitzsimons, J. T. (1966). Hypovolaemic drinking and renin. *J. Physiol. (Lond.)* **186**, 130–131P.

Fitzsimons, J. T. (1969). The role of a renal thirst factor in drinking induced by extracellular stimuli. *J. Physiol. (Lond.)* **201**, 349–368.

Fitzsimons, J. T. and Simons, B. J. (1968). The effect of angiotensin on drinking in the rat. *J. Physiol. (Lond.)* **196**, 34–41P.

Fitzsimons, J. T. and Simons, B. J. (1969). The effect on drinking in the rat of intravenous infusion of angiotensin, given alone or in combination with other stimuli of thirst. *J. Physiol. (Lond.)* **203**, 45–57.

Fletcher, A. and Pradhan, S. N. (1969). Responses to microinjections of *d*-tubocurarine into the hypothalamus of cats. *Int. J. Neuropharmacol.* **8**, 373–377.

Fonnum, F. (1969a). Isolation of choline esters from aqueous solutions by extraction with sodium tetraphenylboron in organic solvents. *Biochem. J. (Lond.)* **113**, 291–293.

Fonnum, F. (1969b). Radiochemical micro assays for the determination of choline acetyltransferase and acetylcholinesterase activities. *Biochem. J. (Lond.)* **115**, 465–472.

Fonnum, F. (1970). Topographical and subcellular localization of choline acetyltransferase in rat hippocampal region. *J. Neurochem.* **17**, 1029–1037.

Forrer, G. R. (1951). Atropine toxicity in the treatment of mental disease. *Amer. J. Psychiat.* **108**, 107–112.

Fragner, J. (1965). "Vitamine" Bd. II, VEB, G. Fischer, Jena.

Frazier, D. T. and Boyarsky, L. L. (1964). Evidence for cholinergic transmission at a central synapse. *Proc. Soc. Exp. Biol. Med.* **115**, 876–879.

Frazier, D. T. and Boyarsky, L. L. (1967). Cholinergic properties of the relay junctions of the primary afferent pathway. *J. Pharmacol. Exp. Therapeut.* **156**, 1–11.

Freedman, A. M. and Himwich, H. E. (1949). DFP: Site of injection and variation in response. *Amer. J. Physiol.* **156**, 125–128.

French, J. D., Verzeano, M. and Magoun, H. W. (1953). A neural basis of the anesthetic state. *Archs. Neurol. Psychiat.* **69**, 519–529.

Fried, P. A. (1972). The Septum and behaviour: A review. *Psychol. Bull.* **78**, 292–310.

Friedman, A. H. and Everett, G. M. (1964). Pharmacological aspects of parkinsonism. *In* "Advances in Pharmacology", pp. 83–127. (S. Garattini and P. A. Shore, Eds) Vol. 3, Academic Press, New York and London.

Friedman, A. H. and Walker, C. A. (1969). Rat brain amines, blood histamine and glucose levels in relationship to circadian changes in sleep induced by pentobarbital sodium. *J. Physiol. (Lond.)* **202**, 133–146.

Friedman, A. H. and Walker, C. A. (1972). The acute toxicity of drugs acting at cholinoceptive sites and twenty-four hour rhythms in brain acetylcholine. *Arch. Toxikol.* **29**, 39–49.

Fulton, J. F. (1951). "Frontal Lobotomy and Affective Behavior". W. W. Norton and Co. Inc., New York, 159 pp.

Fuxe, K. and Hanson, L. C. F. (1967). Central catecholamine neurons and conditioned avoidance behaviour. *Psychopharmacologia* **11**, 439–447.

Fuxe, K. Hökfelt, T. and Ungerstedt, U. (1969). Distribution of monoamines in the mammalian central nervous system by histochemical studies. *In* "Metabolism of Amines in the Brain", pp. 10–22. (G. Hooper, Ed.) Macmillan, London.

Gaddum, J. H. (1961). Push-pull cannulae. *J. Physiol. (Lond.)* **155**, 1P.

Garattini, S., Giacalone, E. and Valzelli, L. (1969). Biochemcical changes during isolation-induced aggressiveness in mice. *In* "Aggressive Behaviour", pp. 179–187. (S. Garattini and E. B. Sigg, Eds) Excerpta Medica Fdn., Amsterdam.

Gardiner, J. E. (1961). The inhibition of acetylcholine synthesis in brain by hemicholinium. *Biochem. J. (Lond.)* **81**, 297–303.

Gastaut, H. (1958). The role of the reticular formation in establishing conditioned reactions. *In* "Reticular Formation of the Brain", pp. 561–590. (H. H. Jasper, L. D. Proctor, R. S. Knighton, W. C. Noshay and R. T. Costello, Eds) Little, Brown and Co., Boston.

Gerard, R. W. (1949). Physiology and psychiatry. *Amer. J. Psychiat.* **106**, 161–173.

Gerebtzoff, M. A. (1959). "Cholinesterases. A Histochemical Contribution to the Solution of Some Functional Problems", 543 pp. Vol. 3, Pergamon Press, Oxford.

Gesell, R. and Hansen, E. T. (1945). Anticholinesterase activity of acid as a biological instrument of nervous integration. *Amer. J. Physiol.* **144**, 126–163.

Gesell, R., Hansen, E. T. and Worzniak, J. J. (1943). Humoral intermediation of nerve cell activation in the central nervous system. *Amer. J. Physiol.* **138**, 776–791.

Giarman, N. J. and Pepeu, G. (1962). Drug-induced changes in brain acetylcholine. *Brit. J. Pharmacol.* **19**, 226–234.

Giarman, N. J. and Pepeu, G. (1964). The influence of centrally acting cholinolytic drugs on brain acetylcholine levels. *Brit. J. Pharmacol. Chemother.* **23**, 123–130.

Ginsberg, B. E. and Allee, W. C. (1942). Some effects of conditioning on social dominance and subordination in inbred strains of mice. *Physiol. Zool.* **15**, 485–506.

Girgis, M. (1973). Histochemical localization of acetylcholinesterase enzyme in the "limbic system" of the brain of the cebus monkey (*Cebus apella*). *Acta Anat.* **84**, 202–223.

Gisselson, L. (1952). The effect of acetylcholine-esterase-inhibiting substances on the muscles of the middle ear and on the latency of the cochlear potentials. *Acta Oto-lar.* **42**, 208–218.

Glassman, E. (1969). The biochemistry of learning: An evaluation of the role of RNA and protein. *Ann. Rev. Biochem.* **38**, 605–646.

Glees, P. and Griffith, H. B. (1952). Bilateral destruction of the hippocampus (*cornu ammonis*) in a case of dementia. *Monatsschr. Psychiat. Neurol.* **123**, 193–204.

Glick, S. D., Mittag, T. W. and Green, J. P. (1973). Central cholinergic correlates of impaired learning. *Neuropharmacology* **12**, 291–296.

Glickman, S. E. (1961). Perseverative neural processes and consolidation of the memory trace. *Psychol. Bull.* **58**, 218–233.

Globus, A., Rosenzweig, M. R., Bennett, E. L. and Diamond, M. C. (1972). Effects of differential experience on dendritic spine counts in rat cerebral cortex. *Int. J. Neurosci.* **4**, 124–129.

Globus, A. and Scheibel, A. B. (1967). The effect of visual deprivation on cortical neurons. *Exp. Neurol.* **19**, 331–345.

Goldberg, A. M. and McCaman, R. E. (1967). A quantitative microchemical study of choline acetyltransferase and acetylcholinesterase in the cerebellum of several species. *Life Sci.* **6**, 1493–1500.

Goldberg, M. E. and Johnson, H. E. (1964). Potentiation of chlorpromazine-induced behavioral changes by anticholinesterase agents. *J. Pharm. Pharmacol.* **16**, 60–61.

Goldberg, M. E., Johnson, H. E. and Knaak, J. B. (1965). Inhibition of discrete avoidance behavior by three anticholinesterase agents. *Psychopharmacologia* **7**, 72–76.

Goldberg, M. E., Johnson, H. E., Knaak, J. B. and Smyth, H. F. Jr., (1963). Psychopharmacological effects of reversible cholinesterase inhibition induced by N-methyl-3-isopropyl phenyl carbamate (compound 10854). *J. Pharmacol. Exp. Therapeut.* **141**, 244–252.

Goldstein, M., Anagnoste, B., Owen, W. S. and Battista, A. F. (1966). The effects of ventromedial tegmental lesions on the biosynthesis of catecholamines in the striatum. *Life Sci.* **5**, 2171–2176.

Gomulicki, B. R. (1953). The development and present status of the trace theory of memory. *Brit. J. Psychol. Monograph Suppl.* **29**, 1–94.

Grace, J. E. (1968). Central nervous system lesions and saline intake in the rat. *Physiol. Behav.* **3**, 387–393.

Graham, D. T. and Erickson, C. K. (1971). The effect of ethanol on the output of cerebral acetylcholine *in vivo*. *Fed. Proc.* **30**, 622.

Granit, R. (1970). "The Basis of Motor Control", 346 pp. Academic Press, New York and London.

Granit, R., Haase, J. and Rutledge, L. T. (1960). Recurrent inhibition in relation to frequency of firing and limitation of discharge rate of extensor motoneurones. *J. Physiol. (Lond.)* **154**, 308–328.

Granit, R., Pascoe, J. E. and Steg, G. (1957). The behaviour of tonic α and γ moto-neurones during stimulation of recurrent collaterals. *J. Physiol. (Lond.)* **138**, 381–400.

Granit, R. and Renkin, B. (1961). Net depolarization and discharge rate of moto-neurones, as measured by recurrent inhibition, *J. Physiol. (Lond.)* **158**, 461-475.

Granit, R. and Rutledge, L. T. (1960). Surplus excitation in reflex action of motoneurones as measured by recurrent inhibition. *J. Physiol. (Lond.)* **154**, 288–307.

Green, J. D. (1960). The hippocampus. *In* "Handbook of Physiology", pp. 1373–1389. (J. Field, Ed.) Vol. II, Section I, American Physiological Society, Washington, D.C.

Green, J. D. and Shimamoto, T. (1953). Hippocampal seizures and their propagation. *Archs. Neurol. Psychiat.* **70**, 687–702.

Green, E. G. (1968). Cholinergic stimulation of medial septum. *Psychonom. Sci.* **10**, 157–158.

Greene, E. G. and Lomax, P. (1970). Impairment of alternation learning in rats following microinjection of carbachol into the hippocampus. *Brain Res.* **18**, 355–359.

Grewal, R. S., Lu, F. C. and Allmark, M. G. (1962). The release of posterior pituitary hormone in the rat by nicotine and lobeline. *J. Pharmacol. Exp. Therapeut.* **135**, 84–88.

Grossman, S. P. (1960). Eating or drinking elicited by direct adrenergic or cholinergic stimulation of hypothalamus. *Science, N.Y.* **132**, 301–302.

Grossman, S. P. (1962a). Direct adrenergic and cholinergic stimulation of hypo-thalamic mechanisms. *Amer. J. Physiol.* **202**, 872–882.

Grossman, S. P. 1962b). Effects of adrenergic and cholinergic blocking agents on hypothalamic mechanisms. *Amer. J. Physiol.* **202**, 1230–1236.

Grossman, S. P. (1964). Behavioral effects of direct chemical stimulation of central nervous system structures. *Int. J. Neuropharmacol.* **3**, 45–58.

Grossman, S. P. (1966a). The VMH: A center for affective reactions, satiety, or both? *Physiol. Behav.* **1**, 1–10.

Grossman, S. P. (1966b). Acquisition and performance of avoidance responses during chemical stimulation of the midbrain reticular formation. *J. Comp. Physiol. Psychol.* **61**, 42–49.

Grossman, S. P. (1968). Behavioral and electroencephalographic effects of micro-injections of neurohumors into the midbrain reticular formation. *Physiol. Behav.* **3**, 777–786.

Grossman, S. P. and Grossman, L. (1966). Effects of chemical stimulation of the mid-brain reticular formation on appetitive behavior. *J. Comp. Physiol. Psychol.* **61**, 333–338.

Grossman, S. P. and Peters, R. (1966). Acquisition of appetitive and avoidance habits following atropine-induced blocking of the thalamic reticular formation. *J. Comp. Physiol. Psychol.* **61**, 325–332.

Grossman, S. P., Peters, R., Freedman, P. and Willer, H. (1965). Behavioral effects of cholinergic stimulation of the thalamic reticular formation. *J. Comp. Physiol. Psychol.* **59**, 57–65.

Gubler, C. J. (1968). Enzyme studies in thiamine deficiency. *Int. Z. Vitam.* **38**, 287–303.

Guerrero-Figueroa, R., Verster, F. De B., Barros, A. and Heath, R. G. (1964). Choli-nergic mechanisms in subcortical mirror focus and effects of topical application of γ-aminobutyric acid and acetylcholine. *Epilepsia* **5**, 140–155.

Guth, L. (1962). Neuromuscular function after regeneration of interrupted nerve fibers into partially denervated muscle. *Exp. Neurol.* **6**, 129–141.

Guth, P. S. and Amaro, J. (1969). A possible cholinergic link in olivo-cochlear inhibi-tion. *Int. J. Neuropharmacol.* **8**, 49–53.

Hadžović, S., Nikolin, B. and Stern, P. (1965). The effect of tremorine and lysergic acid diethylamide on the iron content of the rat brain. *J. Neurochem.* **12,** 908–909.

Hadžović, S., Potkonjak, D. and Stern, P. (1966). Acetylcholine content in different areas of dog's brain after administration of tremorine. *Bull. Sci.*, Sect. A, **11,** 63–64.

Hamburg, M. D. (1967). Retrograde amnesia produced by intraperitoneal injection of physostigmine. *Science, N.Y.* **156,** 973–974.

Hamilton, L. W., Kelsey, J. E. and Grossman, S. P. (1970). Variations in behavioral inhibition following different septal lesions in rats. *J. Comp. Physiol. Psychol.* **70,** 79–86.

Hamilton, L. W., McCleary, R. A. and Grossman, S. P. (1968). Behavioral effects of cholinergic septal blockade in the cat. *J. Comp. Physiol. Psychol.* **66,** 563–568.

Hammar, C. -G., Hanin, I., Holmstedt, B., Kitz, R. J., Jenden, D. J. and Karlén, B. (1968). Identification of acetylcholine in fresh rat brain by combined gas chromatography-mass spectrometry. *Nature (Lond.)* **220,** 915–917.

Hampson, J. L., Essig, C. F., McCauley, A. and Himwich, H. E. (1950). Effects of di-isopropyl fluorophosphate (DFP) on electroencephalogram and cholinesterase activity. *EEG Clin. Neurophysiol.* **2,** 41–48.

Hanin, I. (1969). A specific gas chromatographic method for assaying tissue acetylcholine: Present status. *In* "Advances in Biochemistry and Psychopharmacology", pp. 111–130. (E. Costa and P. Greengaard, Eds) Vol. 1, Raven Press, New York.

Hanin, I., Massarelli, R. and Costa, E. (1970). Acetylcholine concentrations in rat brain: Diurnal oscillation. *Science, N.Y.* **170,** 341–342.

Hanson, H. M., Stone, C. A. and Witoslawski, J. J. (1970). Antagonism of the anti-avoidance effects of various agents by anticholinergic drugs. *J. Pharmacol. Exp. Therapeut.* **173,** 117–124.

Hanson, L. C. F. (1967). Evidence that the central action of (+) amphetamine is mediated via catecholamines. *Psychopharmacologia* **10,** 289–297.

Harlow, H. F. (1965). Sexual behaviour in the rhesus monkeys. *In* "Sex and Behavior", pp. 234–265. (F. A. Beach, Ed.) Wiley, New York.

Harlow, H. F., Dodsworth, R. O. and Harlow, M. K. (1965). Total social isolation in monkeys. *Proc. Nat. Acad. Sci., N.Y.* **54,** 90–96.

Harlow, H. F. and Harlow, M. K. (1962). The effect of rearing conditions on behavior, *Bull. Menninger Clinic* **26,** 213–224.

Harlow, H. F., Harlow, M. K., Dodsworth, R. O. and Arling, G. L. (1966). Maternal behavior of rhesus monkeys deprived of mothering and peer associations in infancy. *Proc. Amer. Phil. Soc.* **110,** 58–66.

Harvey, J. A. and Hunt, H. F. (1965). Effect of septal lesions on thirst in the rat as indicated by water consumption and operant responding for water reward. *J. Comp. Physiol. Psychol.* **59,** 49–56.

Hayward, J. N. and Vincent, J. D. (1970). Osmosensitive single neurones in the hypothalamus of unanaesthetized monkeys. *J. Physiol. (Lond.)* **210,** 947–972.

Hebb, C. O. (1961). Cholinergic neurones in vertebrates. *Nature (Lond.)* **192,** 527–529.

Hebb, C. O. (1963). Formation, storage and liberation of acetylcholine. *Handb. Exp. Pharmak.* **15,** 55–88.

Hebb, C. O. (1970). CNS at the cellular level: Identity of transmitter agents. *Ann. Rev. Physiol.* **32,** 165–192.

Hebb, C. O. and Krnjević, K. (1962). The physiological significance of acetylcholine. *In* "Neurochemistry", pp. 452–521. (K. A. C. Elliott, I. H. Page and J. H. Quastel, Eds) 2nd Ed., C. C. Thomas, Springfield, Illinois.

Hebb, C. O., Krnjević, K. and Silver, A. (1963). Effect of undercutting on the acetyl-cholinesterase and choline acetyltransferase activity in the cat's cerebral cortex. *Nature (Lond.)* **198,** 692.

Hebb, C. O. and Morris, D. (1969). Identification of acetylcholine and its metabolism in nervous tissue. *In* "The Structure and Function of Nervous Tissue", pp. 25–60. (G. H. Bourne, Ed.) Vol. III, Academic Press, London and New York.

Hebb, C. O. and Silver, A. (1956). Choline acetylase in the central nervous system of man and some other mammals. *J. Physiol. (Lond.)* **134,** 718–728.

Hebb, C. O. and Silver, A. (1970). *In* "An Introduction to Neuropathology: Method and Diagnosis", pp. 665–690. (C. G. Tedeschi, Ed.) Little, Brown and Co., Boston.

Hebb, D. O. (1949). "The Organization of Behavior". Wiley, New York.

Hebb, D. O. (1955). Drives and the C.N.S. (conceptual nervous system). *Psychol. Rev.* **62,** 243–254.

Hebb, D. O. (1958). The motivating effects of exteroceptive stimulation. *Amer. Psychol.* **13,** 109–113.

Heilbronn, E. (1970). Further experiments on the uptake of acetylcholine and atropine and the release of acetylcholine from mouse brain cortex slices after treatment with phospholipases. *J. Neurochem.* **17,** 381–389.

Heinrich, C. P., Stadler, H. and Weiser, H. (1973). The effect of thiamine deficiency on the acetylcoenzyme A and acetylcholine levels in the rat brain. *J. Neurochem.* **21,** 1273–1281.

Hemsworth, B. A. and Mitchell, J. F. (1969). The characteristics of acetylcholine mechanisms in the auditory cortex. *Brit. J. Pharmacol. Chemother.* **36,** 161–170.

Hemsworth, B. A. and Neal, M. J. (1968). The effect of central stimulant drugs on acetylcholine release from rat cerebral cortex. *Brit. J. Pharmacol. Chemother.* **34,** 543–550.

Henderson, W. R. and Wilson, W. C. (1936). Intraventricular injections of acetyl-choline and eserine in man. *Quart. J. Exp. Physiol.* **26,** 83–95.

Hendler, N. H. and Blake, W. D. (1969). Hypothalamic implants of angiotensin II, carbachol, and norepinephrine on water and NaCl solution intake in rats. *Commun. Behav. Biol.* **4,** 41–48.

Hensel, H. (1973). Neural processes in thermoregulation. *Physiol. Rev.* **53,** 948–1017.

Heriot, J. T. and Coleman, P. D. (1962). The effect of electroconvulsive shock on retention of a modified "one-trial" conditioned avoidance. *J. Comp. Physiol. Psychol.* **55,** 1082–1084.

Hernández-Peón, R. (1965). Central neuro-humoral transmission in sleep and wake-fulness. *Progr. Brain. Res.,* **18,** 96–117.

Hernández-Peón, R. and Chávez-Ibarra, G. (1963a). Sleep induced by electrical or chemical stimulation of the forebrain. *In* "The Physiological Basis of Mental Acti-vity" (R. Hernández-Peón, Ed.) *EEG Clin. Neurophysiol. Suppl.* **24,** 188–198.

Hernández-Peón, R., Chávez-Ibarra, G., Morgane, P. J. and Timo-Iaria, C. (1963b). Limbic cholinergic pathways involved in sleep and emotional behavior. *Exp. Neurol.* **8,** 93–111.

Heron, W. (1961). Cognitive and physiological effects of perceptual isolation. *In* "Sensory Deprivation", pp. 1–33. (P. Solomon, P. E. Kubzansky, P. H. Leiderman, J. H. Mendelson, R. Trumbull and D. Wexlor, Eds) Harvard University Press, Cambridge.

Herz, A. (1970). Synaptic transmitter substances and seizures. *Pharmakopsychiat. Neuropsychopharmacol.* **3,** 133–150.

Hess, W. R. (1949). "Das Zwischenhirn: Syndrome, Lokalisationen, Funktionen". Schwabe, Basel.

Hess, W. R. (1954). The diencephalic sleep centre. *In* "Brain Mechanisms and Consciousness". (J. F. Delafresnaye, Ed.) C. C. Thomas, Springfield, Illinois.

Hess, W. R. (1957). "The Functional Organization of the Diencephalon". Grune and Stratton, New York.

Hess, W. R. and Brugger, M. (1943). Das subkortikale Zentrum der affektiven Abwehrreaktion. *Helv. Physiol. Pharmacol. Acta* **1**, 35–52.

Hiebel, G., Bonvallet, M., Huve, P. and Dell, P. (1954). Analyse neurophysiologique de l'action central de la *d*-amphetamine (Maxiton). *Semaine des Hôpiteaux de Paris* **30**, 1880–1887.

Hilding, D. and Wersall, J. (1962). Cholinesterase and its relation to the nerve endings in the inner ear. *Acta Oto-lar. Stockh.* **55**, 205–217.

Hilgard, E. R. and Marquis, D. G. (1940). "Conditioning and Learning". Appleton, New York.

Himwich, H. E. (1953). Some effects of DFP and atropine on behavior. *Arzneimittelforsch.* **3**, 228–231.

Himwich, H. E., Essig, C. F., Hampson, J. L., Bales, P. D. and Freedman, A. M. (1950). Effect of trimethadione (Tridione) and other drugs on convulsions caused by di-isopropyl fluorophosphate (DFP). *Amer. J. Psychiat.* **106**, 816–820.

Hoffer, A. (1954). Induction of sleep by autonomic drugs. *J. Nerve Ment. Dis.* **119**, 421–427.

Holmstedt, B. (1959). Pharmacology of organophosphorus cholinesterase inhibitors. *Pharmacol. Rev.* **11**, 567–688.

Holmstedt, B. and Lundgren, G. (1966). Tremorogenic agents and brain acetylcholine. *In* "Mechanisms of Release of Biogenic Amines", pp. 439–468. (U.S. von Euler, S. Rosell and B. Uvnas, Eds) Pergamon Press, Oxford.

Holmstedt, B., Lundgren, G. and Sundwall, A. (1963). Tremorine and atropine effects on brain acetylcholine. *Life Sci.* **10**, 731–736.

Hornykiewics, O. (1960). Dopamine (3-hydroxytyramine) and brain function. *Pharmacol. Rev.* **18**, 925–964.

Hosein, E. A., Chabrol, J. G. and Freedman, G. (1966). Effect of thiamine deficiency in rats and pigeons on content of materials with acetylcholine-like activity in brain, heart and skeletal muscle. *Rev. Can. Biol.* **25**, 129–134.

Hosein, E. A., Proulx, P. and Ara, R. (1962). Substances with acetylcholine activity in normal rat brain. *Biochem. J. (Lond.)* **83**, 341–346.

Houser, V. P. and Houser, F. L. (1973). The effects of agents that modify muscarinic tone upon behavior controlled by an avoidance schedule that employs signaled unavoidable shock. *Psychopharmacologia* **32**, 133–150.

Huang, J. J. (1938). A vagus-post-pituitary reflex. *Chin. J. Physiol.* **13**, 367–382.

Hubbard, J. I. (1961). The effect of calcium and magnesium on the spontaneous release of transmitter from mammalian motor nerve terminals. *J. Physiol. (Lond.)* **159**, 507–517.

Hubbard, J. I., Jones, S. F. and Landau, E. M. (1968). On the mechanism by which calcium and magnesium affect the spontaneous release of transmitter from mammalian motor nerve terminals. *J. Physiol. (Lond.)* **194**, 355–380.

Hull, C. D., Buchwald, N. A. and Ling, G. (1967). Effects of direct cholinergic stimulation of forebrain structures. *Brain Res.* **6**, 22–35.

Hunsperger, R. W. (1956). Affektreaktionen auf elektrische Reizung im Hirnstamm der Katze. *Helv. Physiol. Pharmacol. Acta* **14**, 70–92.

Hymovich, B. (1952). The effects of environmental variations on problem solving in the rat. *J. Comp. Physiol. Psychol.* **45**, 313–321.

Igić, R., Jeličić, J. and Stern, P. (1968). Oxotremorine activity in beri-beri pigeons. *Pharmacology* **1**, 161–164.

Igić, R. and Stern, P. (1971). The effect of oxotremorine on the free and bound brain acetylcholine concentrations and motor activity in beri-beri pigeons. *Can. J. Physiol. Pharmacol.* **49**, 985–987.

Igić, R., Stern, P. and Basagić, E. (1970). Changes in emotional behaviour after application of cholinesterase inhibitor in the septal and amygdala region. *Neuropharmacology* **9**, 73–75.

Ilyutechenok, R. I. (1962). The role of cholinergic systems of the brainstem reticular formation in the mechanism of central effects of anticholinesterase and cholinolytic drugs. *In* "Pharmacological Analysis of Central Nervous Action", pp. 211–216. (W. D. M. Paton, Ed.) Vol. 8, Macmillan, New York.

Israël, M. and Whittaker, V. P. (1965). The isolation of mossy fiber endings from the granular layer of the cerebellar cortex. *Experientia* **21**, 325–326.

Izquierdo, J. A., Baratti, C. M., Torrelio, M., Arévalo, L. and McGaugh, J. L. (1973). Effects of food deprivation, discrimination experience and physostigmine on choline acetylase and acetylcholine esterase in the dorsal hippocampus and frontal cortex of rats. *Psychopharmacologia* **33**, 103–110.

Izquierdo, I. and Izquierdo, J. A. (1971). Effects of drugs on deep brain centers. *Ann. Rev. Pharmacol.* **11**, 189–208.

Jasper, H. H. (1949). Diffuse projection systems: The integrative action of the thalamic reticular system. *EEG Clin. Neurophysiol.* **1**, 405–420.

Jasper, H. H. (1958). Recent advances in our understanding of ascending activities of the reticular system. *In* "Reticular Formation of the Brain", pp. 319–331. (H. H. Jasper L. D. Proctor, R. S. Knighton, W. C. Noshay and R. T. Costello, Eds) Henry Ford Hosp. Int. Symp., Little, Brown and Co., Boston.

Jasper, H. H., Ajmone-Marsan, C. and Stoll, J. (1952). Corticofugal projections to the brain stem. *Archs. Neurol. Psychiat. (Chic.)* **67**, 155–171.

Jasper, H. H. and Koyama, I. (1967). Rate of release of acetylcholine and glutamic acid from the cerebral cortex during reticular activation. *Fed. Proc.* **26**, 373.

Jasper, H. H. and Koyama, I. (1968). Amino acids released from the cortical surface in cats following stimulation of the mesial thalamus and midbrain reticular formation. *EEG Clin. Neurophysiol.* **24**, 292.

Jasper, H. H. and Koyama, I. (1969). Rate of release of amino acids from the cerebral cortex in the cat as affected by brainstem and thalamic stimulation. *Can. J. Physiol. Pharmacol.* **47**, 889–905.

Jasper, H. H. and Tessier, J. (1971). Acetylcholine liberation from cerebral cortex during paradoxical (REM) sleep. *Science, N.Y.* **172**, 601–602.

Jasser, A. and Guth, P. S. (1973). The synthesis of acetylcholine by the olivo-cochlear bundle. *J. Neurochem.* **20**, 45–53.

Jennings, R. (1963). Modification of maze learning in rats by posttrial injections of atropine or physostigmine. Unpublished Ph.D. thesis, University of Colorado.

Jenny, E. H. and Healy, S. T. (1959). Drug antagonists to chlorpromazine inhibition of the conditioned response. *Fed. Proc.* **18**, 407.

Jhamandas, K., Pinsky, C. and Phillis, J. W. (1970). Effects of morphine and its antagonists on release of cerebral cortical acetylcholine. *Nature (Lond.)* **228**, 176–177.

Jhamandas, K., Pinsky, C. and Phillis, J. W. (1971). Effects of narcotic analgesics and antagonists on the *in vivo* release of acetylcholine from the cerebral cortex of the cat. *Brit. J. Pharmacol. Chemother.* **43**, 53–66.

Jouvet, E. R. (1967). "Mechanisms of Memory". 468 pp. Academic Press, London and New York.

Jordan, L. M. and Phillis, J. W. (1972). Acetylcholine inhibition in the intact and chronically isolated cerebral cortex. *Brit. J. Pharmacol. Chemother.* **45**, 584–595.

Jouvet, M. (1961). Telencephalic and rhombencephalic sleep in the cat. *In* "Ciba Fdn. Symp., Nature of Sleep", pp. 188–206. (G. E. Wolstenholme and M. O'Connor, Eds) Churchill, London.

Jouvet, M. (1965). Paradoxical sleep—A study of its nature and mechanisms. *Progr. Brain Res.* **18**, 20–62.

Jouvet, M. (1967). Neurophysiology of sleep. *In* "The Neurosciences", pp. 529–544. (G. C. Quarton, T. Melnechuk and F. O. Schmitt, Eds) Rockefeller University Press, New York.

Jouvet, M. (1969). Biogenic amines and the states of sleep. *Science, N.Y.* **163**, 32–41.

Jung, O. H. and Boyd, E. S. (1966). Effects of cholinergic drugs on self-stimulation response rates in rats. *Amer. J. Physiol.* **210**, 432–434.

Kalyuzhnyi, L. V. (1962). Food and defensive conditioned reflexes in rabbits after injection of norepinephrine and carbachol into hypothalamus. *Zhurnal Vysshei Nervnoĭ Deiatel' nosti* **12**, 318.

Kanai, T. and Szerb, J. C. (1965). Mesencephalic reticular activating system and cortical acetylcholine output. *Nature (Lond.)* **205**, 80–82.

Kandel, E. R. and Spencer, W. A. (1968). Cellular neurophysiological approaches in the study of learning. *Physiol. Rev.* **48**, 65–134.

Kao, C. V. (1966). Tetrodotoxin, saxitoxin and their significance in the study of excitation phenomena. *Pharmacol. Rev.* **18**, 997–1049.

Karczmar, A. G. (1967). Pharmacologic, toxicologic, and therapeutic properties of anticholinesterase agents. *In* "Physiological Pharmacology", pp. 163–322. Vol. III (W. S. Root and F. G. Hoffmann, Eds) Academic Press, London and New York.

Karczmar, A. G. (1969). Is the central cholinergic nervous system overexploited? *Fed. Proc.* **28**, 147–157.

Karli, P. (1956). The Norway rat's killing response to the white mouse. *Behaviour* **10**, 81–103.

Kása, P., Joó, F. and Csillik, B. C. (1965). Histochemical localization of acetylcholinesterase in the cat cerebellar cortex. *J. Neurochem.* **12**, 31–35.

Kása, P., Mann, S. P. and Hebb, C. O. (1970a). Localization of choline acetyltransferase—Histochemistry at the light microscope level. *Nature (Lond.)* **226**, 812–814.

Kása, P., Mann, S. P. and Hebb, C. O. (1970b). Localization of choline acetyltransferase—Ultrastructural localization in spinal neurones. *Nature (Lond.)* **226**, 814–816.

Kása, P. and Silver, A. (1969). The correlation between choline acetyltransferase and acetylcholinesterase activity in different areas of the cerebellum of rat and guinea pig. *J. Neurochem.* **16**, 389–396.

Kasé, Y. and Borison, H. L. (1958). Central respiratory depressant action of "hemicholinium" in the cat. *J. Pharmacol. Exp. Therapeut.* **122**, 215–233.

Kawamura, H. and Domino, E. F. (1968). Hippocampal slow ("arousal") wave activation in the rostral midbrain transected cat. *EEG Clin. Neurophysiol.* **25**, 471–480.

Kawamura, H. and Domino, E. F. (1969). Differential actions of *m* and *n* cholinergic agonists on the brainstem activating system. *Int. J. Neuropharmacol.* **8**, 105–115.

Kawamura, H., Nakamura, Y. and Tokizane, T. (1961). Effects of acute brainstem lesions on the electrical activity of the neocortex and the limbic system. *Jap. J. Physiol.* **11**, 564–575.

Khavari, K. A. (1971). Adrenergic-cholinergic involvement in modulation of learned behavior. *J. Comp. Physiol. Psychol.* **74**, 284–291.

Khavari, K. A. and Maickel, R. P. (1967). Atropine and atropine methylbromide effects on behavior of rats. *Int. J. Neuropharmacol.* **6**, 301–306.

Kiernon, J. A. (1964). Carboxylic esterases of the hypothalamus and neurohypophysis of the hedgehog. *J. Roy. Micr. Soc.* **83**, 297–306.

Killam, E. K. (1962). Drug action on the brainstem reticular formation. *Pharmacol. Rev.* **14**, 175–223.

Killam, K. F. and Killam, E. K. (1958). Drug action on pathways involving the reticular formation. In "Reticular Formation of the Brain", pp. 111–122. (H. H. Jasper, L. D. Procter, R. S. Knighton, W. C. Noshay and R. T. Costello, Eds) Henry Ford Hosp. Int. Symp., Little, Brown and Co., Boston.

King, C. D. and Jewett, R. E. (1971). The effects of methyltyrosine on sleep and brain norepinephrine in cats. *J. Pharmacol. Exp. Therapeut.* **177**, 188–195.

King, F. A. (1958). Effects of septal and amygdaloid lesions on emotional behavior and conditioned avoidance responses in the rat. *J. Nerv. Ment. Dis.* **126**, 57–63.

Kirkpatrick, W. E. and Lomax, P. (1970). Temperature changes following iontophoretic injection of acetylcholine into the rostral hypothalamus of the rat. *Neuropharmacology* **9**, 195–202.

Klawans, H. L. (1968). The pharmacology of parkinsonism (a review). *Dis. Nerv. Syst.* **29**, 805–817.

Klüver, H. and Bucy, P. C. (1937). "Psychic blindness" and other symptoms following bilateral temporal lobectomy in Rhesus monkeys. *Amer. J. Physiol.* **119**, 352–353.

Klüver, H. and Barerra, E. (1953). A method for the combined staining of cells and fibers in the nervous system. *J. Neuropath. Exp. Neurol.* **12**, 400–403.

Knapp, D. E. and Domino, E. F. (1962). Action of nicotine on the ascending reticular activating system. *Int. J. Neuropharmacol.* **1**, 333–351.

Koelle, G. B. (1969). Significance of acetylcholinesterase in central synaptic transmission. *Fed. Proc.* **28**, 95–100.

Koelle, G. B. and Geesey, C. N. (1961). Localization of acetylcholinesterase in the neurohypophysis and its functional implications. *Proc. Soc. Exp. Biol. Med.* **106**, 625–628.

Konorski, J. (1948). "Conditioned Reflexes and Neuron Organization". Cambridge University Press, New York, and Cambridge.

Kooy, F. H. (1919). Hyperglycemia in mental disorders. *Brain* **17**, 214.

Krech, D., Rosenzweig, M. R. and Bennett, E. L. (1960). Effects of environmental complexity and training on brain chemistry. *J. Comp. Physiol. Psychol.* **53**, 509–519.

Krech, D., Rosenzweig, M. R. and Bennett, E. L. (1962a). Relations between brain chemistry and problem solving among cats raised in enriched and impoverished environments. *J. Comp. Physiol. Psychol.* **55**, 801–807.

Krech, D., Rosenzweig, M. R. and Bennett, E. L. (1962b). Effects of environmental complexity and training on brain chemistry. *J. Comp. Physiol. Psychol.* **53**, 509–519.

Krech, D., Rosenzweig, M. R. and Bennett, E. L. (1963). Effects of complex environment and blindness on rat brain. *Archs. Neurol. (Chic.)* **8**, 403–412.

Krech, D., Rosenzweig, M. R. and Bennett, E. L. (1966). Environmental impoverishment, social isolation and changes in brain chemistry and anatomy. *Physiol. Behav.* **1**, 99–104.

Kremer, M. (1942). Action of intrathecally injected prostigmine, acetylcholine, and eserine on the central nervous system in man. *Quart. J. Exp. Physiol.* **31**, 337–357.

Krikstone, B. J. and Levitt, R. A. (1970). Interactions between water deprivation and chemical brain stimulation. *J. Comp. Physiol. Psychol.* **71**, 334–340.

Krnjević, K. (1964). Micro-iontophoretic studies on cortical neurones. *Int. Rev. Neurobiol.* **7**, 41–98.

Krnjević, K. (1965a). Actions of drugs on single neurones in the cerebral cortex. *Brit. Med. Bull.* **21**, 10–14.

Krnjević, K. (1965b). Cholinergic innervation of the cerebral cortex. *In* "Studies in Physiology", pp. 144–151. (D. R. Curtis and A. K. McIntyre, Eds) Springer, Berlin.

Krnjević, K. (1967). Chemical transmission and cortical arousal. *Anesthesiology* **28**, 100–105.

Krnjević, K. (1969). Central cholinergic pathways. *Fed. Proc.* **28**, 113–120.

Krnjević, K. and Phillis, J. W. (1963a). Acetylcholine-sensitive cells in the cerebral cortex. *J. Physiol. (Lond.)* **166**, 296–327.

Krnjević, K. and Phillis, J. W. (1963b). Pharmacological properties of acetylcholine-sensitive cells in the cerebral cortex. *J. Physiol. (Lond.)* **166**, 328–350.

Krnjević, K. and Phillis, J. W. (1963c). Iontophoretic studies of neurones in the mammalian cerebral cortex. *J. Physiol. (Lond.)* **165**, 274–304.

Krnjević, K. and Silver, A. (1965). A histochemical study of cholinergic fibres in the cerebral cortex. *J. Anat. (Lond.)* **99**, 711–759.

Kuhar, M. J., Sethy, V. H., Roth, R. H. and Aghajanian, G. K. (1973). Choline: Selective accumulation by central cholinergic neurons. *J. Neurochem.* **20**, 581–593.

Kumagai, H., Sakai, F. and Otsuka, Y. (1962). Analysis of the central effect of d-tubocurarine chloride in the cat. *Int. J. Neuropharmacol.* **1**, 157–159.

Kuno, M. and Rudomin, P. (1966). The release of acetylcholine from the spinal cord of the cat by antidromic stimulation of motor nerves. *J. Physiol. (Lond.)* **187**, 177–193.

Kuriyama, K., Roberts, E. and Vos, J. (1968). Some characteristics of binding of $\gamma$-aminobutyric acid and acetylcholine to a synaptic vesicle fraction from mouse brain. *Brain Res.* **9**, 231–252.

Kurokawa, M., Kato, M. and Machiyama, Y. (1961). Choline acetylase activity in a convulsive strain of mouse. *Biochim. Biophys. Acta* **50**, 385–386.

Kurokawa, M., Naruse, H. and Kato, M. (1966). Metabolic studies on *ep* mouse, a special strain with convulsive predisposition. *Progr. Brain Res.* **21A**, 112–130.

Lalley, P. M., Rossi, G. V. and Baker, W. W. (1970). Analysis of local cholinergic tremor mechanisms following selective neurochemical lesions. *Exp. Neurol.* **27**, 258–275.

Lamarre, Y. and Cordeau, J. P. (1963). Central unit activity in monkeys with postural tremor. *Fed. Proc.* **22**, 1771.

Larochelle, L., Bédard, P., Poirier, L. J. and Sourkes, T. L. (1971). Correlative neuroanatomical and neuropharmacological study of tremor and catatonia in the monkey. *Neuropharmacology* **10**, 273–288.

Leaf, R. C. and Muller, S. A. (1966). Central cholinergic response inhibition during massed free-operant and discrete-trial avoidance acquisition. *In* "Proc. Fifth Int. Congr. Collegium Int. Neuro-Psycho-Pharm". Excerpta Medica Fdn., Amsterdam.

Lederis, K. (1962). The distribution of vasopressin and oxytocin in hypothalamic nuclei. *In* "Neurosecretion", pp. 227–235. (H. Heller and R. B. Clark, Eds) Pergamon Press, London.

Lederis, K. and Livingston, A. (1966). Acetylcholine content in the rabbit neurohypophysis. *J. Physiol. (Lond.)* **185**, 37–38.

Lederis, K. and Livingston, A. (1969). Acetylcholine and related enzymes in the neural lobe and anterior hypothalamus of the rabbit. *J. Physiol. (Lond.)* **201**, 695–709.

Lefresne, P., Guyenet, P. and Glowinski, J. (1973) Acetylcholine synthesis from [2-$^{14}$C] pyruvate in rat striatal slices. *J. Neurochem.* **20**. 1083–1097.

Lehmann, A. (1970). Relationship between sympathetic ganglion activity and audiogenic seizures in mice. *Life Sci.* (Part I) **9**, 251–257.

Leibowitz, S. F. and Miller, N. E. (1969). Unexpected adrenergic effect of chlorpromazine: Eating elicited by injection into rat hypothalamus. *Science, N.Y.* **165**, 609–611.

Levinson, P. K. and Flynn, J. P. (1965). The objects attacked by cats during stimulation of the hypothalamus. *Anim. Behav.* **13**, 217–220.

Levitt, R. A. (1970). Temporal decay of the blockade of carbachol drinking by atropine. *Physiol. Behav.* **5**, 627–628.

Levitt, R. A. and Boley, R. P. (1970). Drinking elicited by injection of eserine or carbachol into rat brain. *Physiol. Behav.* **5**, 693–695.

Levitt, R. A. and Buerger, P. B. (1970). Interactions between cholinergic mechanisms and the salt arousal of drinking. *Learning and Motiva.* **1**, 297–303.

Levitt, R. A. and Fisher, A. E. (1966). Anticholinergic blockade of centrally induced thirst. *Science, N.Y.* **154**, 520–522.

Levitt, R. A., White, C. S. and Sander, D. M. (1970). Dose-response analysis of carbachol-elicited drinking in the rat limbic system. *J. Comp. Physiol. Psychol.* **72**. 345–350.

Lewis, P. R. and Shute, C. C. D. (1967). The cholinergic limbic system: Projection to hippocampal formation, medial cortex, nucleus of ascending cholinergic reticular system and subfornical organ and supra-optical crest. *Brain* **90**, 521–540.

Lewis, P. R., Shute, C. C. D. and Silver, A. (1967). Confirmation from choline acetylase analysis of massive cholinergic innervation of the rat hippocampus. *J. Physiol. (Lond.)* **191**, 215–224.

Lindsley, D. B. (1951). Emotion *In* "Handbook of Experimental Psychology", pp. 473–516. (S. S. Stevens, Ed.) Wiley, New York.

Lindsley, D. B. (1957). Psychophysiology and motivation. *In* "Nebraska Symp. on Motivation", pp. 44–105. (M. R. Jones, Ed.) University of Nebraska Press, Lincoln.

Linét, O., Widhalm, S. and Heartting, G. (1967). The influence of experimental thiamine-avitaminosis on catecholamine levels in hearts and brains of pigeons. *Int. J. Neuropharmacol.* **6**, 337–339.

Livingston, R. B. (1955). Some brain stem mechanisms relating to psychosomatic functions. *Psychosomat. Med.* **17**, 347–354.

Lomax, P. and Jenden, D. J. (1966). Hypothermia following systemic and intracerebral injection of oxotremorine in the rat. *Neuropharmacology* **5**, 353–359.

Long, J. P. (1963). Structure-activity relationships of the reversible anticholinesterase agents. *In* "Cholinesterases and Anticholinesterase Agents" pp. 374–427 (G. B. Koelle, Ed.) Handbuch der Experimentellen Pharmakologie, Vol. 15, Springer-Verlag, Berlin.

Long, J. P. and Schueler, F. W. (1954). A new series of cholinesterase inhibitors. *J. Amer. Pharm. Assoc. Sci. Ed.* **43**, 79–86.

Longo, V. G. (1966). Mechanism of the behavioral and electroencephalographic effects of atropine and related compounds. *Pharmacol. Rev.* **18**, 965–996.

Longo, V. G. and Scotti de Carlos, A. (1968). Anticholinergic hallucinogenics: Laboratory results *versus* clinical trials. *Progr. Brain Res.* **28**, 106–112.

Lorente de Nó, R. (1938). Analysis of the activity of the chains of internuncial neurons. *J. Neurophysiol.* **1**, 207–244.

Lovett, D. and Singer, G. (1971). Ventricular modification of drinking and eating behavior. *Physiol. Behav.* **6**, 23–26.

Lundgren, G. and Malmburg, M. (1968). Effects of oxotremorine on brain acetylcholine formation *in vivo* and *in vitro*. *Biochem. Pharmacol.* **17**, 2051–2056.

MacDonnell, M. F. and Flynn, J. P. (1966a). Control of sensory fields by stimulation of hypothalamus. *Science, N.Y.* **152**, 1406–1408.

MacDonnell, M. F. and Flynn, J. P. (1966b). Sensory control of hypothalamic attack. *Anim. Behav.* **14**, 399–405.

MacIntosh, F. C. (1941). The distribution of acetylcholine in the peripheral and the central nervous system. *J. Physiol. (Lond.)* **99**, 436–442.

MacIntosh, F. C. (1963). Synthesis and storage of acetylcholine in nervous tissue. *Can. J. Biochem. Physiol.* **41**, 2555–2571.

MacIntosh, F. C. and Oborin, P. E. (1953). Release of acetylcholine from intact cerebral cortex. *Abstr. XIX Int. Physiol. Congr.* pp. 580–581.

MacLean, P. D. (1949). Psychosomatic disease and the "visceral brain". Recent developments bearing on the Papez theory of emotion. *Psychosom. Med.* **11**, 338–353.

MacLean, P. D. (1957). Chemical and electrical stimulation of the hippocampus in unrestrained animals. I. Methods and electroencephalographic findings. *Archs. Neurol. Psychiat.* **78**, 113–127.

MacLean, P. D. (1958). Contrasting functions of limbic and neocortical systems of the brain and their relevance to psychophysiological aspects of medicine. *Amer. J. Med.* **25**, 611–626.

MacLean, P. D. and Delgado, J. M. R. (1953). Electrical and chemical stimulation of frontotemporal portion of limbic system in the waking animal. *EEG Clin. Neurophysiol.* **5**, 91–100.

Magoun, H. W. (1954). The ascending reticular system and wakefulness. *In* "Brain Mechanisms and Consciousness", pp. 1–20. (J. F. Delafresnaye, Ed.) C. C. Thomas, Springfield, Illinois.

Mah, C. J. and Albert, D. J. (1973). Electroconvulsive shock-induced retrograde amnesia: An analysis of the variation in the length of the amnesia gradient. *Behav. Biol.* **9**, 517–540.

Maickel, R. P., Stern, D. N. and Brodie, B. B. (1964). *In* "Proc. Second Int. Pharmacol. Meeting", Vol. 2, pp. 225–237. Pergamon Press, Oxford.

Mann, P. J. G., Tennenbaum, M. and Quastel, J. H. (1939). Acetylcholine metabolism in the central nervous system; the effects of potassium and other cations on acetylcholine liberation. *Biochem. J. (Lond.)* **33**, 822–835.

Mann, S. A. (1925). Blood-sugar studies in mental disorders. *J. Ment. Sci.* **71**, 443–482.

Marchbanks, R. M. (1969). Biochemical organization cholinergic nerve terminals in the cerebral cortex. "Symposium International Society Cell Biology", pp. 115–135. Vol. 8, Academic Press, London and New York.

Mason, W. A. (1963). Social development of rhesus monkeys with restricted social experience. *Motor Skills* **16**, 263–270.

Matsuda, T., Hata, F. and Yoshida, H. (1968). Stimulatory effect of $Na^+$ and ATP on the release of acetylcholine from synaptic vesicles. *Biochim. Biophys. Acta* **150**, 739–741.

McCaman, R. E. and Hunt, J. M. (1965). Microdetermination of choline acetylase in nervous tissue. *J. Neurochem.* **12**, 253–259.

McCance, I. and Phillis, J. W. (1964a). The action of acetylcholine on cells in cat cerebellar cortex. *Experientia* **20**, 217–218.

McCance, I. and Phillis, J. W. (1964b). The discharge patterns of elements in cat cerebellar cortex and their responses to iontophoretically applied drugs. *Nature (Lond.)* **204**, 844–846.

McCance, I. and Phillis, J. W. (1968). Cholinergic mechanisms in the cerebellar cortex. *Int. J. Neuropharmacol.* **7**, 447–462.

McCance, I., Phillis, J. W. and Westerman, R. A. (1968). Acetylcholine-sensitivity of thalamic neurones: Its relationship to synaptic transmission. *Brit. J. Pharmacol. Chemother.* **32**, 635–651.

McCandless, D. W. and Schenker, S. (1968). Encephalopathy of thiamine deficiency: Studies of intracerebral mechanisms. *J. Clin. Invest.* **47**, 2268–2280.

McCleary, R. A. (1961). Response specificity in the behavioral effects of limbic system lesions in the cat. *J. Comp. Physiol. Psychol.* **54**, 605–613.

McCleary, R. A. (1966). Response-modulating functions of the limbic system: Initiation and suppression. *In* "Progress in Physiological Psychology". (E. Stellar and J. M. Sprague, Eds) Vol. 1, Academic Press, New York and London.

McGaugh, J. L. (1966). Time-dependent processes in memory storage. *Science, N.Y.* **153**, 1351–1358.

McGaugh, J. L. (1968). Drug facilitation of memory and learning. *In* "Psychopharmacology: A Review of Progress, 1957–1967" (D. A. Efron J. O. Cole, J. Levine and J. R. Whittenborn, Eds) U.S. Publ. Health Serv. Public No. 1836, pp. 891–904.

McGaugh, J. L. and Petrinovich, L. (1959). The effect of strychnine sulphate on maze learning. *Amer. J. Psychol.* **72**, 99–102.

McGaugh, J. L. and Petrinovich, L. (1965). Effects of drugs on learning and memory. *Int. Rev. Neurobiol.* **8**, 139–196.

McGaugh, J. L. and Thomson, C. W. (1962). Facilitation of simultaneous discrimination learning with strychnine sulphate. *Psychopharmacologia* **3**, 166–172.

McGeer, E. G., Wada, S. A., Terao, A. and Jung, E. (1969). Amine synthesis in various brain regions with caudate or septal lesions. *Exp. Neurol.* **24**, 277–284.

McKim, W. A. (1973). The effects of scopolamine on fixed-interval behaviour in the rat: A rate-dependency effect. *Psychopharmacologia* **32**, 255–264.

McKinney, T. D. (1970). Brain cholinesterase in grouped and singly caged adrenal-demedullated rats. *Amer. J. Physiol.* **219**, 331–334.

McLennan, H. (1964). The release of acetylcholine and of 3-hydroxytyramine from the caudate nucleus. *J. Physiol. (Lond.)* **174**, 152–161.

Méhes, J. (1929). Studien über den Skopolaminschlaf und seine Verstarkung durch Morphium. *Arch. Exp. Path. Pharmakol.* **142**, 309–322.

Meissner, W. W. (1966). Special review. Hippocampal functions in learning. *J. Psychiat. Res.* **4**, 235–304.

Mennear, J. H. (1965). Interactions between central cholinergic agents and amphetamine in mice. *Psychopharmacologia* **7**, 107–114.

Metz, B. (1956). A respiratory reflex as affected by an anticholinesterase. *Amer. J. Physiol.* **185**, 142–144.

Metz, B. (1958). Brain acetylcholinesterase and a respiratory reflex. *Amer. J. Physiol.* **192**, 101–105.

Metz, B. (1961). The brain ACh-AChE-ChA system in respiratory control. *Neurology (Minneap.)* **11**, 37–45.

Metz, B. (1962). Correlation between respiratory reflex and acetylcholine content of pons and medulla. *Amer. J. Physiol.* **202**, 80–82.

Metz, B. (1964). High arterial $pCO_2$, low pH, the ACh-AChE system in the medulla, and respiratory activity. *Neurology (Minneap.)* **14**, 425–433.

Metz, B. (1966). Hypercapnia and acetylcholine release from the cerebral cortex and medulla. *J. Physiol. (Lond.)* **186**, 321–332.

Metz, B. (1969). Release of ACh from the carotid body by hypoxia and hypoxia plus hypercapnia. *Resp. Physiol.* **6**, 386–394.

Metz, B. (1971a). Correlation between the electrical activity and acetylcholine release from the cerebral cortex and medulla during hypercapnia. *Can. J. Physiol. Pharmacol.* **49**, 331–337.

Metz, B. (1971b). Acetylcholine and experimental brain injury. *J. Neurosurg.* **35**, 523–528.

Meyers, B. (1965). Some effects of scopolamine on a passive avoidance response in rats. *Psychopharmacologia* **8**, 111–119.

Michaelis, M., Arango, N. I. and Gerard, R. W. (1949). Inhibition of brain dehydrogenases by "anticholinesterases". *Amer. J. Physiol.* **157**, 463–467.

Mihkelson, M. J. (1961). Pharmacological evidences of the role of acetylcholine in the higher nervous activity of man and animals. *Activ. Nerv. Sup.* **3,** 140–147.

Miller, F. R., Stavraky, G. W. and Woonton, G. A. (1940). Effects of eserine, acetylcholine and atropine on electrical corticogram. *J. Neurophysiol.* **3,** 131–138.

Miller, J. J. (1956). Symposium on atropine toxicity therapy; pharmacology procedure and techniques in atropine toxicity treatment of mental illnesses. *J. Nerv. Ment. Dis.* **124,** 260–264.

Miller, N. E. (1960). Motivational effects of brain stimulation and drugs. *Fed. Proc.* **19,** 846–854.

Miller, N. E. (1965). Chemical coding of behavior in the brain. *Science, N.Y.* **148,** 328–338.

Miller, N. E., Bailey, C. J. and Stevenson, J. A. F. (1950). Decreased "hunger" but increased food intake resulting from hypothalamic lesions. *Science, N.Y.* **112,** 256–259.

Miller, N. E. and Chien, C. -W. (1968). Drinking elicited by injecting eserine into preoptic area of rat brain. *Commun. Behav. Biol.* **1,** 61–63.

Miller, N. E., Gottesman, K. S. and Emery, N. (1964). Dose response to carbachol and norepinephrine in rat hypothalamus. *Amer. J. Physiol.* **206,** 1384–1388.

Minz, B. and Agid, R. (1937). Influence de la vitamine B$_1$ sur l'activité de l'acétylcholine. *C.R. Acad. Sci. Paris.* **205,** 576–580.

Mitchell, J. F. (1960). Release of acetylcholine from the cerebral cortex and the cerebellum. *J. Physiol. (Lond.)* **155,** 22–23P.

Mitchell, J. F. (1963). The spontaneous and evoked release of acetylcholine from the cerebral cortex. *J. Physiol. (Lond.)* **165,** 98–116.

Mitchell, J. F. (1966). Acetylcholine release from the brain. In "Mechanisms of Release of Biogenic Amines, Proc. Wenner-Gren Symp.", pp. 425–437. Pergamon Press, Oxford.

Mitchell, J. F. and Phillis, W. J. (1962). Cholinergic transmission in the frog spinal cord. *Brit. J. Pharmacol. Chemother.* **19,** 534–543.

Mitchell, J. F. and Szerb, J. C. (1962). The spontaneous and evoked release of acetylcholine from the caudate nucleus. *Abstr. XXII Int. Physiol. Congr.*, No. 819.

Molenaar, P. C. and Polak, R. L. (1970). Stimulation by atropine of acetylcholine release and synthesis in cortical slices from rat brain. *Brit. J. Pharmacol. Chemother.* **40,** 406–417.

Molnár, J. György, L., Pfeiffer, K. A. and Nádor, K. (1967). Tremorigenic and convulsant actions of intracerebrally administered vegetative poisons in the mouse. *Acta Physiol. Acad. Sci. Hung.* **31,** 249–256.

Monnier, M. (1959). Stimulants hallucinogènes, psychotoniques et analeptiques du système nerveux central. *Abstr. Symp. XXI Int. Physiol. Congr., Buenos Aires*, p. 149.

Morgan, M. J. (1973). Effects of post-weaning environment on learning in the rat. *Anim. Behav.* **21,** 429–442.

Morgane, P. J. (1964). Limbic-hypothalamic-midbrain interaction in thirst and thirst motivated behavior. In "Thirst", pp. 429–455. (M. J. Wayner, Ed.) Pergamon Press, Oxford.

Morpurgo, C. and Theobald, W. (1964). Influence of antiparkinson drugs and amphetamine on some pharmacological effects of phenothiazine derivatives used as neuroleptics. *Psychopharmacologia* **6,** 178–191.

Moruzzi, G. and Magoun, H. W. (1949). Brain stem reticular formation and activation of the EEG. *E.E.G. Clin. Neurophysiol.* **1,** 455–473.

Moss, R. L., Urban, I. and Cross, B. A. (1972). Microelectrophoresis of cholinergic and aminergic drugs on paraventricular neurons. *Amer. J. Physiol.* **223,** 320–318.

Moyer, K. E. (1968). Kinds of aggression and their physiological basis. *Commun. Behav. Biol.* **2,** 65–87.

Mulas, A. and Pepeu, G. (1970). Disappearance in rats with septal lesions of the stimulatory effect of hyoscine on exploratory behaviour. *Brit. J. Pharmacol. Chemother.* **39**, 209P.

Myers, R. D. (1964). Emotional and autonomic responses following hypothalamic chemical stimulation. *Can. J. Psychol.* **18**, 6–14.

Myers, R. D. (1969). Chemical mechanisms in the hypothalamus mediating eating and drinking in the monkey. *Ann. N.Y. Acad. Sci.* **157**, 918–933.

Myers, R. D. and Beleslin, D. B. (1970). The spontaneous release of 5-hydroxytryptamine and acetylcholine within the diencephalon of the unanaesthetized Rhesus monkey. *Exp. Brain Res.* **11**, 539–552.

Myers, R. D. and Sharpe, L. G. (1968). Chemical activation of ingestive and other hypothalamic regulatory mechanisms. *Physiol. Behav.* **3**, 987–995.

Myers, R. D. and Yaksh, T. L. (1968). Feeding and temperature responses in the unrestrained rat after injections of cholinergic and aminergic substances into the cerebral ventricles. *Physiol. Behav.* **3**, 917–928.

Myers, R. D. and Yaksh, T. L. (1969). Control of body temperature in the unanaesthetized monkey by cholinergic and aminergic systems in the hypothalamus. *J. Physiol. (Lond.)* **202**, 483–500.

Nakamura, R., Cheng, S. -C. and Naruse, H. (1970). A study on the precursors of the acetyl moiety of acetylcholine in brain slices. *Biochem. J. (Lond.)* **118**, 443–450.

Narahashi, T., Moore, J. W. and Scott, W. R. (1964). Tetrodotoxin blockage of sodium conductance increase in lobster giant axons. *J. Gen. Physiol.* **47**, 965–974.

Naruse, H., Kato, M., Kurokawa, M., Haba, R. and Yabe, T. (1960). Metabolic defects in a convulsive strain of mouse. *J. Neurochem.* **5**, 359–369.

Nashold, B. S. (1959). Cholinergic stimulation of globus pallidus in man. *Proc. Soc. Exp. Biol. Med.* **101**, 68–69.

Nathan, P., Aprison, M. H. and Himwich, H. E. (1955). A comparison of the effects of atropine with those of several central nervous system stimulants on rabbits exhibiting forced circling following the intracarotid injection of di-isopropyl fluorophosphate. *Confin. Neurol.* **15**, 1–10.

Nauta, W. J. H. (1963). Central nervous organization and the endocrine motor system. *In* "Advances in Neuroendocrinology". (A. R. Nalbondov, Ed.) University of Illinois Press, Urbana, Illinois.

Nauta, W. J. H. and Mehler, W. R. (1966). Projections of the lentiform nucleus in the monkey. *Brain Res.* **1**, 3–42.

Nauta, W. J. H. and Whitlock, D. G. (1954). An anatomical analysis of the non-specific thalamic projection system. *In* "Symp. Brain Mechanisms and Consciousness", pp. 81–98. (J. F. Delafresnaye, Ed.) Blackwell, Oxford.

Navaratnam, V. and Lewis, P. R. (1970). Cholinesterase-containing neurones in the spinal cord of the rat. *Brain Res.* **18**, 411–425.

Neal, M. J., Hemsworth, B. A. and Mitchell, J. F. (1968). The excitation of central cholinergic mechanisms by stimulation of the auditory pathway. *Life Sci.* **7**, (Part I) 757–763.

Nikki, P. (1968). Influence of some cholinomimetic and cholinolytic drugs on halothane shivering in mice. *Ann. Med. Exp. Fenn.* **46**, 521–530.

Nikki, P. (1969). "Pharmacological Studies on Halothane Shivering in Mice and Rats". Mercatorin Kirjapaino, Helsinki.

Nistri, A., Bartolini, A., Deffenu, G. and Pepeu, G. (1972). Investigations into the release of acetylcholine from the cerebral cortex of the cat: Effects of amphetamine, of scopolamine and of septal lesions. *Neuropharmacology* **11**, 665–674.

Norris, C., Guth, P. S. and Stockwell, M. F. (1972). Release of acetylcholine by the olivo-cochlear bundles. *Fed. Proc.* **31**, 580.

Odutola, A. B. (1970). The topographical localization of acetylcholinesterase in the adult rat cerebellum: A reappraisal. *Histochemie* **23**, 98–106.

Olds, J. (1958). Self-stimulation experiments and differentiated reward systems. In "Reticular Formation of the Brain", pp. 671–687. (H. H. Jasper, L. D. Proctor, R. S. Knighton, W. C. Noshay and R. T. Costello, Eds) Little, Brown and Co., Boston.

Olds, J. (1958). Self-stimulation of the brain. *Science, N.Y.* **127**, 315–324.

Olds, J. (1962). Hypothalamic substrates of reward. *Physiol. Rev.* **42**, 554–604.

Olds, M. E. and Domino, E. F. (1969a). Comparison of M and N cholinergic agonists on self-stimulation behavior. *J. Pharmacol. Exp. Therapeut.* **166**, 189–204.

Olds, M. E. and Domino, E. F. (1969b). Differential effects of cholinergic agonists on self-stimulation and escape behavior. *J. Pharmacol. Exp. Therapeut.* **170**, 157–167.

Olds, J. and Milner, P. (1954). Positive reinforcement produced by electrical stimulation of septal area and other regions of rat brain. *J. Comp. Physiol. Psychol.* **47**, 419–427.

Olivier, A., Parent, A., Simard, H. and Poirier, L. J. (1970). Cholinesterasic striato-pallidal and striatonigral efferents in the cat and the monkey. *Brain Res.* **18**, 273–282.

O'Neil, J. J. and Sakimoto, T. (1970). Enzymatic fluorometric determination of acetylcholine in biological extracts. *J. Neurochem.* **17**, 1451–1460.

Ostfeld, A. M. and Aruguete, A. (1962). Central nervous system effects of hyoscine in man. *J. Pharmacol. Exp. Therapeut.* **137**, 133–139.

Ostfeld, A. M., Jenkins, R. and Pasnau, R. (1959). Dose-response data for autonomic and mental effects of atropine and hyoscine. *Fed. Proc.* **18**, 430.

Pakkenberg, H. (1963). Globus pallidus in Parkinsonism. *Acta Neurol. Scand.* **39**, suppl. **4**, 139–144.

Papez, J. W. (1937). A proposed mechanism of emotion. *Archs. Neurol. Psychiat.* **38**, 725–743.

Pasetto, N. (1952). Sul meccanismo colinergico delle ipotalamo postipofisarie. *Arch. Fisiol.* **52**, 1–6.

Pazzagli, A. and Pepeu, G. (1964). Amnesic properties of scopolamine and brain acetylcholine in the rat. *Int. J. Neuropharmacol.* **4**, 291–299.

Penfield, W. and Milner, B. (1958). Memory deficit produced by bilateral lesions in the hippocampal zone. *Archs. Neurol. Psychiat.* **79**, 475–497.

Pepeu, G. (1963). Effect of tremorine and some anti-Parkinson's disease drugs on acetylcholine in the rat's brain. *Nature (Lond.)* **200**, 895.

Pepeu, G. (1972). Cholinergic neurotransmission in the central nervous system. *Arch. Int. Pharmacodyn., suppl.* **196**, 229–243.

Pepeu, G. and Bartolini, A. (1967). Effeto di alcuni psicofarmaci sulla liberazione di acetilcolina dalla corteccia cerebrale di gatto. *Boll. Soc. Ital. Biol. Sper.* **43**, 1409–1412.

Pepeu, G. and Bartolini, A. (1968). Effect of psychoactive drugs on the output of acetylcholine from the cerebral cortex of the cat. *Eur. J. Pharmacol.* **4**, 254–263.

Pepeu, G. and Mantegazzini, P. (1964). Midbrain hemisection: Effect on cortical acetylcholine in the cat. *Science, N.Y.* **145**, 1069–1070.

Pepeu, G., Mulas, A. and Mulas, M. L. (1973). Changes in the acetylcholine content in the rat brain after lesions of the septum, fimbria and hippocampus. *Brain Res.* **57**, 153–164.

Pepeu, G., Mulas, A., Ruffi, A. and Sotgiu, P. (1971). Brain acetylcholine levels in rats with septal lesions. *Life Sci.* **10** (Part I) 181–184.

Petrinovich, L. (1963). Facilitation of successive discrimination learning with strychnine sulphate. *Psychopharmacologia* **4**, 103–113.

Pfeiffer, C. C. (1959). Parasympathetic neurohumors; possible precursors and effect on behavior. *Int. Rev. Neurobiol.* **1**, 195–244.

Pfeiffer, C. C. and Jenny, E. H. (1957). The inhibition of the conditioned response and the counteraction of schizophrenia by muscarinic stimulation of the brain. *Ann. N.Y. Acad. Sci.* **66**, 753–764.

Phillis, J. W. (1965a). Cholinesterase in the cat cerebellar cortex, deep nuclei and peduncles. *Experientia* **21**, 266–268.

Phillis, J. W. (1965b). Cholinergic mechanisms in the cerebellum. *Brit. Med. Bull.* **21**, 26–29.

Phillis, J. W. (1968a). Acetylcholine release from the cerebral cortex: Its role in cortical arousal. *Brain Res.* **7**, 378–389.

Phillis, J. W. (1968b). Acetylcholinesterase in the feline cerebellum. *J. Neurochem.* **15**, 691–698.

Phillis, J. W. (1970). "The Pharmacology of Synapses", 358 pp. Pergamon Press, Oxford.

Phillis, J. W. (1971). The pharmacology of thalamic and geniculate neurons. *Int. Rev. Neurobiol.* **14**, 1–48.

Phillis, J. W. and Chong, G. C. (1965). Acetylcholine release from the cerebral and cerebellar cortices: Its role in cortical arousal. *Nature (Lond.)* **207**, 1253–1255.

Phillis, J. W., Tebécis, A. K. and York, D. H. (1968). Acetylcholine release from the feline thalamus. *J. Pharm. Pharmacol.* **20**, 476–478.

Phillis, J. W. and York, D. H. (1968). Pharmacological studies on a cholinergic inhibition in the cerebral cortex. *Brain Res.* **10**, 297–306.

Pickford, M. (1939). The inhibitory effect of acetylcholine on water diuresis in the dog, and its pituitary transmission. *J. Physiol. (Lond.)* **95**, 226–238.

Pickford, M. (1947). The action of acetylcholine in the supraoptic nucleus of the chloralosed dog. *J. Physiol. (Lond.)* **106**, 264–270.

Pickford, M. (1960). Factors affecting milk release in the dog and the quantity of oxytocin liberated by suckling. *J. Physiol. (Lond.)* **152**, 515–526.

Pickford, M. and Watt, J. A. (1951). A comparison of the effect of intravenous and intracarotid injections of acetylcholine in the dog. *J. Physiol. (Lond.)* **114**, 333–335.

Platt, E. E. (1951). The effects of subcutaneous injection of diisopropyl fluorophosphate (DFP) on the rate of learning a discrimination problem by albino rats. Ph.D. Thesis, Ohio State Univ., Columbus, Ohio.

Poirier, L. J., McGeer, E. G., Larochelle, L., McGeer, P. L., Bédard, P. and Boucher, R. (1969). The effect of brain stem lesions on tyrosine and tryptophan hydroxylases in various structures of the telencephalon of the cat. *Brain Res.* **14**, 147–155.

Poirier, L. J. et Sourkes, T. L. (1964). Influence du *locus niger* sur la concentration des catécholamines du striatum. *J. Physiol. (Paris)* **56**, 426–427.

Poirier, L. J. and Sourkes, T. L. (1965). Influence of the substantia nigra on the catecholamine content of the straitum. *Brain* **88**, 181–192.

Polak, R. L. (1965). Effect of hyoscine on the output of acetylcholine into perfused cerebral ventricles of cats. *J. Physiol. (Lond.)* **181**, 317–323.

Polak, R. L. (1971a). An analysis of the influence of antimuscarinic agents on synthesis, storage and release of acetylcholine by cortical slices from rat brain. Drukkerij De Bij, Amsterdam.

Polak, R. L. (1971b). The stimulating action of atropine on the release of acetylcholine by rat cerebral cortex *in vitro*. *Brit. J. Pharmacol. Chemother.* **41**, 600–606.

Polak, R. L. and Meeuws, M. M. (1966). The influence of atropine on the release and uptake of acetylcholine by the isolated cerebral cortex of the rat. *Biochem. Pharmacol.* **15**, 989–992.

Pope, A., Morris, A. A., Jasper, H., Elliott, K. A. C. and Penfield, W. (1947). Histochemical and action potential studies on epileptogenic areas of cerebral cortex in man and the monkey. *Res. Publ. Assn. Nerv. Ment. Dis.* **26**, 218–231.

Pradhan, S. N., Bhattacharya, I. C. and Atkinson, K. S. (1967). The effects of intraventricular administration of nicotine on blood pressure and some somatic reflexes. *Ann. N.Y. Acad. Sci.* **142**, 50–66.

Pradhan, S. N. and Dutta, S. N. (1971). Central cholinergic mechanism and behavior. *Int. Rev. Neurobiol.* **14**, 173–231.

Prescott, J. W. (1971). Early somatosensory deprivation as an ontogenetic process in the abnormal development of the brain and behavior. *In* "Med. Primatol, Proc. 2nd Conf. Exp. Med. Surg. Primates", pp. 356–375. Karger, Basel.

Proctor, C. D., Ridlon, S. A., Fudema, J. J. and Prabhu, V. G. (1964). Extension of tranquilizer action by anticholinesterases. *Toxicol. Appl. Pharmacol.* **6**, 1–8.

Pryor, G. T., Otis, L. S., Scott, M. K. and Colwell, J. J. (1967). Duration of chronic electroshock treatment in relation to brain weight, brain chemistry and behavior. *J. Comp. Physiol. Psychol.* **63**, 236–239.

Pryor, G. T., Otis, L. S. and Uyeno, E. (1966). Chronic electrochock: Effects on brain weight, brain chemistry and behavior. *Psychonom. Sci.* **4**, 85–86.

Quartermain, D. and Miller, N. E. (1966). Sensory feedback in time-response of drinking elicited by carbachol in preoptic area of the rat. *J. Comp. Physiol. Pholsyc.* **62**, 350–353.

Quastel, J. H. (1962). Acetylcholine distribution and synthesis in the central nervous system. *In* "Neurochemistry", pp. 431–451. (K. A. C. Elliott, I. H. Page and J. H. Quastel, Eds) 2nd Ed., C. C. Thomas, Springfield, Illinois.

Quastel, J. H. (1969). Carbohydrate metabolism in the nervous system. *In* "The Structure and Function of Nervous Tissue", pp. 61–107. (G. H. Bourne, Ed.) Vol. III, Academic Press, London and New York.

Quay, W. B., Bennett, E. L., Rosenzweig, M. R. and Krech, D. (1969). Effects of isolation and environmental complexity on brain and pineal organ. *Physiol. Behav.* **4**, 489–494.

Racine, R. J. and Kimble, D. P. (1965). Hippocampal lesions and delayed alternation in the rat. *Psychonom. Sci.* **3**, 285–286.

Ramwell, P. W., Shaw, J. E. and Jessup, R. (1966). Spontaneous and evoked release of prostaglandins from frog spinal cord. *Amer. J. Physiol.* **211**, 990–1004.

Randić, M. and Padjen, A. (1967). Effect of calcium ions on the release of acetylcholine from the cerebral cortex. *Nature (Lond.)* **215**, 990.

Randić, M. and Straughan, D. W. (1965). Iontophoretic study of paleocortical neurones. *J. Physiol. (Lond.)* **177**, 67–68P.

Randrup, A. and Munkvad, I. (1966). Role of catecholamines in the amphetamine excitatory response. *Nature (Lond.)* **211**, 540.

Rao, K. S., Bhatt, R. H. V., Gopalakrishna, G. and Haranath, P. S. R. K. (1970). Influence of intracarotid infusions of hexamethonium on acetylcholine release from perfused cerebral ventricles in anesthetized dogs. *Indian J. Med. Res.* **58**, 1279–1284.

Ratković, D., Stern, P. and Bošković, B. (1965). Über die Wirkung des Tremorins auf die cholinacetylase. *Bull. Sci.* **10**, 40.

Rech, R. H. (1968). The relevance of experiments involving injection of drugs into the brain. *In* "Importance of Fundamental Principles in Drug Evaluation", pp. 326–360. (D. H. Tedeschi and R. E. Tedeschi, Eds) Raven Press, New York.

Reeves, C. (1966). Cholinergic synaptic transmission and its relationship to behavior. *Psychol. Bull.* **65**, 321–335.

Reimann, C., Lluch, S. and Glick, G. (1972). Development and evaluation of an experimental model for the study of the cerebral circulation in the unanesthetized goat. *Stroke*, **3**, 322–328.

Reis, D. J. (1971). Brain monoamines in aggression and sleep. *Clin. Neurosurg.* **18**, 471–502.

Reitzil, N. L. and Long, J. P. (1959). Hemicholinium antagonism by choline analogues. *J. Pharmacol. Exp. Therapeut.* **127**, 15–21.

Renshaw, B. (1941). Influence of discharge of motoneurons upon excitation of neighbouring motoneurons. *J. Neurophysiol.* **4**, 167–183.

Rheinberger, M. and Jasper, H. (1937). The electrical activity of the cerebral cortex in the unanesthetized cat. *Amer. J. Physiol.* **119**, 186–196.

Richter, D. and Crossland, J. (1949). Variation in acetylcholine content of the brain with physiological state. *Amer. J. Physiol.* **159**, 247–255.

Riesen, A. H. (1966). Sensory deprivation. *In* "Progress in Physiological Psychology". (E. Stellar and J. M. Sprague, Eds) Vol. 1, pp. 117–147. Academic Press, New York and London.

Rimski, B. and Stern, P. (1967). Staticki tremor miseva poslije trovanja disulfidom. *Iugoslav. Physiol. Pharmacol. Acta* **3**, 398.

Rinaldi, F. and Himwich, H. E. (1955a). Alerting responses and actions of atropine and cholinergic drugs. *Archs. Neurol. Psychiat. (Chic.)* **73**, 387–395.

Rinaldi, F. and Himwich, H. E. (1955b). Cholinergic mechanism involved in function of mesodiencephalic activating system. *Archs. Neurol. Psychiat. (Chic.)* **73**, 396–402.

Roa, P. D., Tews, J. K. and Stone, W. E. (1964). A neurochemical study of thiosemicarbazide seizures and their inhibition by aminooxyacetic acid. *Biochem. Pharmacol.* **13**, 477–487.

Roberts, E. and Matthysse, S. (1970). Neurochemistry: At the crossroads of neurobiology. *Ann. Rev. Biochem.* **39**, 777–820.

Rogers, K. T., DeVries, L., Keper, C. R. and Spiedel, E. R. (1960). Studies on chick brain of biochemical differentiation related to morphological differentiation and onset of function. *J. Exp. Zool.*, **144**, 89–103.

Rosecrans, J. A., Dren, A. T. and Domino, E. F. (1968). Effects of physostigmine on rat brain acetylcholine, acetylcholinesterase and conditioned pole jumping. *Int. J. Neuropharmacol.* **7**, 127–134.

Rosenburg, P. and Echlin, F. A. (1968). Time course of changes in cholinesterase activity of chronic partially isolated cortex. *J. Nerv. Ment. Dis.* **147**, 56–64.

Rosenzweig, M. R., Bennett, E. L. and Diamond, M. C. (1967). Cerebral effects of differential experience. "Symp. on Cellular Mechanisms in Learning", *Ann. Meeting Amer. Psychol. Assn., Washington*, D.C.

Rosenzweig, M. R. and Leiman, A. L. (1968). Brain Functions. *Ann. Rev. Psychol.* **19**, 55–98.

Rosenzweig, M. R., Møllgaard, K., Diamond, M. C. and Bennett, E. L. (1972). Theoretical note—Negative as well as positive synaptic changes may store memory. *Psychol. Rev.* **79**, 93–96.

Rossi, G. and Cortesina, G. (1965). The "efferent cochlear and vestibular system" in *Lepus cuniculus L. Acta Anat. (Basel)* **60**, 362–381.

Rossi, G. and Cortesina, G. (1966). Acetylcholinesterase activity in the efferent cochlear fibres after destruction of the organ of corti and afferent fibres. *Acta Oto-lar. Stockh.* **61**, 488–494.

Roth, L. J. (1965). Penetration of drugs into the brain. *In* "Parkinson's Disease", pp. 98–107. (A. Barbeau, L. J. Doshay and E. A. Spiegel, Eds) Grune and Stratton, New York.

Routtenberg, A. (1971). Forebrain pathways of reward in *Rattus norvegicus*. *J. Comp. Physiol. Psychol.* **75**, 269–276.

Rowsell, E. V. (1954). Applied electrical pulses and the ammonia and acetylcholine of isolated cerebral cortex slices. *Biochem. J. (Lond.)* **57**, 666–673.

Rudy, T. A. and Wolf, H. H. (1972). Effect of intracerebral injections of carbamyl-choline and acetylcholine on temperature regulation in the cat. *Brain Res.* **38**, 117–130.

Russell, R. W. (1954). Effects of reduced brain cholinesterase on behavior. *Bull. Brit. Psychol. Soc.* **3**, 6.

Russell, R. W. (1969). Behavioral aspects of cholinergic transmission. *Fed. Proc.* **28**, 121–131.

Russell, R. W., Watson, R. H. J. and Frankenhauser, M. (1961). The effects of chronic reductions in brain cholinesterase activity on the acquisition and extinction of a conditioned avoidance response. *Scand. J. Psychol.* **2**, 21–29.

Ruždik, N. (1965). Promjene tremorinskog efekta pod deistvom intrapalidalno apliciranih supstanci. Postgrad. Thesis, Sarajevo.

Ruždik, N. and Stern, P. (1966). The importance of globus pallidus in the production of rest tremor. *Med. Pharm. Exp. (Basel)* **14**, 17.

Sackett, G. P. (1968). Abnormal behaviour in laboratory reared rhesus monkeys. *In* "Abnormal Behavior in Animals", pp. 293–331. (M. W. Fox, Ed.) Saunders, Philadelphia.

Salmoiraghi, G. C., Bloom, F. E. and Costa, E. (1964). Adrenergic mechanisms in rabbit olfactory bulb. *Amer. J. Physiol.* **207**, 1417–1424.

Salmoiraghi, G. C. and Stefanis, C. N. (1967). A critique of iontophoretic studies of central nervous system neurons. *Int. Rev. Neurobiol.* **10**, 1–30.

Salmoiraghi, G. C. and Steiner, F. A. (1963). Acetylcholine sensitivity of cat's medullary neurons. *J. Neurophysiol* **26**, 581–597.

Saunders, V. F. (1966). Effect of behavioral and environmental manipulations on central ChE activity in the rat. *Fed. Proc.* **25**, 1102.

Scheel-Krüger, J. (1970). Central effects of anticholinergic drugs measured by the apomorphine gnawing test in mice. *Acta Pharmacol. Toxicol* **28**, 1–16.

Scheibel, M. E. and Scheibel, A. B. (1966). Spinal motoneurons, interneurons and Renshaw cells. A Golgi study. *Archs. Ital. Biol.* **104**, 328–353.

Schelkunov, E. L. (1967). Integrated effect of psychotropic drugs on the balance of cholino-, adreno-, and serotoninergic processes in the brain as a basis of their gross behavioural and therapeutic actions. *Activ. Nerv. Sup. (Praha)* **9**, 207–217.

Schildkraut, J. J. and Kety, S. S. (1967). Biogenic amines and emotion. *Science, N.Y.* **156**, 21–30.

Schlosberg, H. (1954). Three dimensions of emotion. *Psychol. Rev.* **61**, 81–88.

Schuberth, J., Sollenberg, J., Sundwall, A. and Sorbo, B. (1966). Acetyl-coenzyme A in brain. The effect of centrally active drugs, insulin coma and hypoxia. *J. Neurochem.* **13**, 819–822.

Schueler, F. W. (1955). A new group of respiratory paralyzants. I. The "hemicholiniums". *J. Pharmacol. Exp. Therapeut.* **115**, 127–143.

Schueler, F. W. (1960). The mechanism of action of the hemicholiniums. *Int. Rev. Neurobiol.* **2**, 77–97.

Schuh, F. (1970). On the binding of diisopropyl-phosphoro-fluoridate (DFP) to plasma proteins. *Arch. Toxikol.* **26**, 262–272.

Schuknecht, H. F. (1958). Acetylcholinesterase and the olivo-cochlear tract of Rasmussen. *Laryngoscope (St. Louis)* **68**, 627.

Schuknecht, H. F., Churchill, J. A. and Doran, R. (1959). The localization of acetyl-cholinesterase in the cochlea. *A.M.A. Archs. Otolar* **69**, 549–559.

Schweikart, G. E. and Collins, G. (1966). The effects of differential postweaning environments on later behavior in the rat. *J. Genet. Psychol.* **109**, 255–263.

Schweitzer, A. and Wright, S. (1938). Action of nicotine on the spinal cord. *J. Physiol. (Lond.)* **94**, 136–147.

Scoville, W. B. and Milner, B. (1957). Loss of recent memory after bilateral hippocampal lesions. *J. Neurol. Neurosurg. Psychiat.* **20**, 11–21.

Sethy, V. H., Kuhar, M. J., Roth, R. H., Van Woert, M. H. and Aghajanian, G. K. (1973). Cholinergic neurons: Effect of acute septal lesions on acetylcholine and choline content of rat hippocampus. *Brain Res.* **55**, 481–484.

Severs, W. B. and Daniels-Severs, A. E. (1973). Effects of angiotensin on the central nervous system. *Pharmacol. Rev.* **25**, 415–449.

Sharpe, L. G. and Myers, R. D. (1969). Feeding and drinking following stimulation of the diencephalon of the monkey with amines and other substances. *Exp. Brain Res.* **8**, 295–310.

Sherwood, S. L. (1952). Intraventricular medication in catatonic stupor. *Brain* **75**, 68–75.

Shopsin, B., Stern, S. and Gershon, S. (1972). Altered carbohydrate metabolism during treatment with lithium carbonate. *Archs. Gen. Psychiat.* **26**, 566–571.

Shute, C. C. D. and Lewis, P. R. (1961). *Bibl. Anat. (Basel)* **2**, 34 (Cited by Storm-Mathisen, 1970).

Shute, C. C. D. and Lewis, P. R. (1963). Cholinesterase-containing systems of the brain of the rat. *Nature (Lond.)* **199**, 1160–1164.

Shute, C. C. D. and Lewis, P. R. (1965). Cholinesterase-containing pathways of the hindbrain: Afferent cerebellar and centrifugal cochlear fibres. *Nature (Lond.)* **205**, 242–246.

Shute, C. C. D. and Lewis, P. R. (1967). The ascending cholinergic reticular system: Neocortical, olfactory and subcortical projections. *Brain* **90**, 497–520.

Sie, G., Jasper, H. H. and Wolfe, L. S. (1965). Rate of ACh release from cortical surface in *encephale* and *cerveau isolé* cat preparations in relation to arousal and epileptic activation of the ECoG. *EEG Clin. Neurophysiol.* **18**, 206.

Silver, A. (1967). Cholinesterases of the central nervous system with special reference to the cerebellum. *Int. Rev. Neurobiol.* **10**, 57–109.

Skinner, B. F. (1953). "Science and Human Behavior". Macmillan, New York.

Slangan, J. L. and Miller, N. E. (1969). Pharmacological tests for the function of hypothalamic norepinephrine in eating behavior. *Physiol. Behav.* **4**, 543–552.

Smelik, P. G. and Ernst, A. M. (1966). Role of nigro-neostriatal dopaminergic fibers in the compulsive gnawing behavior in rats. *Life. Sci.* **5**, 1485–1488.

Smith, D. E., King, M. B. and Hoebel, B. G. (1970). Lateral hypothalamic control of killing: Evidence for a cholineceptive mechanism. *Science, N.Y.* **167**, 900–901.

Smith, O. A. (1956). Stimulation of lateral and medial hypothalamus and food intake in the rat. *Anat. Rec.* **124**, 363–364.

Snell, R. S. (1961). The histochemical localization of cholinesterase in the central nervous system. *Bibl. Anat. (Basel)* **2**, 50–58.

Snider, R. S. (1950). Recent contributions to the anatomy and physiology of the cerebellum. *Archs. Neurol. Psychiat.* **64**, 196–219.

Sollberger, A. (1960). Studies of temporal variations in biological variates. *Suppl. Rep. 5th Int. Conf. Soc. Biol. Rhythm.* Stockholm, 111 pp.

Sollberger, A. (1965). "Biological Rhythm Research", 481 pp. Elsevier, Amsterdam.

Sommer, S. R., Novin, D. and Levine, M. (1967). Food and water intake after intrahypothalamic injections of carbachol in the rabbit. *Science, N.Y.* **156**, 983–984.

Sorensen, J. P., Jr. and Harvey, J. A. (1971). Decreased brain acetylcholine after septal lesions in rats; correlation with thirst. *Physiol. Behav.* **6**, 723–725.

Sotgiu, P., Ruffi, A. and Pepeu, P. (1971). Behavioural effects caused by intra-arterial injection of acetylcholine and nicotine in conscious rats. *Pharmacol. Res. Commun.* **3**, 45–53.

Spatz, H. (1922). Über den Eisennachweis im Gehirn, besonders in Zentren des extrapyramidal-motorischen Systems. *Z. Ges. Neurol. Psychiat.* **77**, 261.

Speeg, K. V., Chen, D., McCandless, D. W. and Schenker, S. (1970). Cerebral acetylcholine in thiamine deficiency. *Proc. Soc. Exp. Biol. Med.* **134**, 1005–1009.

Spiegel, E. A., Wycis, H. T., Marks, M. and Lee, A. J. (1947). Stereotaxic apparatus for operations on the human brain. *Science, N.Y.* **106**, 349–350.

Spitz, R. A. (1945). Hospitalism, an inquiry into the genesis of psychiatric conditions in early childhood. *Psychoanal. Stud. Child.* **1**, 53–74.

Squire, L. R. (1970). Physostigmine: Effects on retention at different times after brief training. *Psychonom. Sci.* **19**, 49.

Squire, L. R., Glick, S. D. and Goldfarb, J. (1971). Relearning at different times after training as affected by centrally and peripherally acting cholinergic drugs in the mouse. *J. Comp. Physiol. Psychol.* **74**, 41–45.

Stadler, H., Lloyd, K. G., Gadea-Ciria, M. and Bartolini, G. (1973). Enhanced striatal acetylcholine release by chlorpromazine and its reversal by apomorphine. *Brain Res.* **55**, 476–480.

Stark, P. and Boyd, E. S. (1963). Effects of cholinergic drugs on hypothalamic self-stimulation response rates in dogs. *Amer. J. Physiol.* **205**, 745–748.

Starzl, T. E. and Magoun, H. W. (1951). Organization of the diffuse thalamic projection system. *J. Neurophysiol.* **14**, 133–146.

Starzl, T. E., Taylor, C. W. and Magoun, H. W. (1951). Collateral afferent excitation of the reticular formation of the brain stem. *J. Neurophysiol.* **14**, 479–496.

Stavinoha, W. B. and Ryan, L. C. (1965). Estimation of the acetylcholine content of rat brain by gas chromatography. *J. Pharmacol. Exp. Therapeut.* **150**, 231–235.

Stein, L. (1969). *In* "Reinforcement and Behavior", pp. 328–355. (J. T. Tapp, Ed.) Academic Press, New York and London.

Stein, L. and Seifter, J. (1962). Muscarinic synapses in the hypothalamus. *Amer. J. Physiol.* **202**, 751–756.

Stern, P. (1964). Ueber die Uebertragungssubstanz der Renshawzellen. *Naturwiss.* **51**, 90–91.

Stern, P. and Gašparović, I. (1962). "Proc. 1st Int. Pharmacol. Meeting", p. 149. Pergamon Press, Oxford.

Stern, P., Hadžović, S. and Nikolin, B. (1966). Bedeutung des Eisens im Corpus striatum für den Tremor. *Naunyn-Schmiedebergs Arch. Pharmak. Exp. Path.* **257**, 67.

Stern, P. and Hasanagić, E. (1967). The influence of oxotremorine on the level of total flavines in the rat brain. *J. Neurochem.* **14**, 1129–1132.

Stern, P., Hasanagić, E. and Fuks, Ž. (1969). The influence of oxotremorine on iron and flavines in mitochondria from rat brain corpus striatum. *Biochem. Pharmacol.* **18**, 940–942.

Stern, P. and Igić, R. (1970). *In* "Drugs and Cholinergic Mechanisms in the CNS", p. 419. (E. Heilbronn and A. Winter, Eds) Stockholm.

Stevens, J. R., Portland, O., Chul, K., Seoul, K. and MacLean, P. D. (1961). Stimulation of the caudate nucleus. *Archs. Neurol. (Chic.)* **4**, 47–54.

Stevens, R. J. (1973). A cholinergic inhibitory system in the frog optic tectum; its role in visual electrical responses and feeding behavior. *Brain Res.* **49**, 309–321.

Stevenson, J. A. F. (1964). The hypothalamus in the regulation of energy and water balance. *Physiologist* **7**, 305–318.

Stone, T. W. (1972). Cholinergic mechanisms in the rat somatosensory cerebral cortex. *J. Physiol. (Lond.)* **225**, 485–499.

Stone, W. E. (1957). The role of acetylcholine in brain metabolism and function. *Amer. J. Phys. Med.* **36**, 222–255.

Storm-Mathisen, J. (1970). Quantitative histochemistry of acetylcholinesterase in rat hippocampal region correlated to histochemical staining. *J. Neurochem.* **17**, 739–750.

Storm-Mathisen, J. and Fonnum, F. (1969). Neurotransmitter synthesis in excitatory and inhibitory synapses of rat hippocampus. *Abstr. Second Int. Meeting, Int. Soc. Neurochem.*, Milan, p. 382.

Stratton, L. O. and Petrinovich, L. (1963). Post-trial injections of an anti-cholinesterase drug and maze learning in two strains of rats. *Psychopharmacologia* **5**, 47–54.

Stricker, E. M. (1966). Extracellular fluid volume and thirst. *Amer. J. Physiol.* **211**, 232–238.

Stümpf, Ch. (1965). Drug action on the electrical activity of the hippocampus. *Int. Rev. Neurobiol.* **8**, 77–138.

Szabo, J. (1962). Topical distribution of the striatal efferents in the monkey. *Exp. Neurol.* **5**, 21–36.

Szerb, J. C. (1963). Nature of acetylcholine-like activity released from brain *in vivo*. *Nature (Lond.)* **197**, 1016–1017.

Szerb, J. C. (1964). The effect of tertiary and quaternary atropine on cortical acetylcholine output and on the electroencephalogram in cats. *Can. J. Physiol. Pharmacol.* **42**, 303–314.

Szerb, J. C. (1967). Cortical acetylcholine release and electroencephalographic arousal. *J. Physiol. (Lond.)* **192**, 329–343.

Szerb, J. C., Malik, H. and Hunter, E. G. (1970). Relationship between acetylcholine content and release in the cat's cerebral cortex. *Can. J. Physiol. Pharmacol.* **48**, 780–790.

Szerb, J. C. and Somogyi, G. T. (1973). Depression of acetylcholine release from cerebral cortical slices by cholinesterase inhibition and by oxotremorine. *Nature (Lond.)* **241**, NB 121–122.

Timsit, J. (1966). Sur l'activité cataleptique de quelques dérivés de la butyrophénone. *Therapie* **21**, 1453–1471.

Tobias, J. M., Lipton, M. A. and Lepinat, A. A. (1946). Effect of anaesthetics and convulsants on brain-acetylcholine content. *Proc. Soc. Exp. Biol. Med.* **61**, 51–54.

Torii, S. and Wikler, A. (1965). Effects of atropine on electrical activity of neocortex and hippocampus in cat. *Fed. Proc.* **24**, 516.

Tower, D. B. and Elliott, K. A. C. (1952). Activity of acetylcholine systems in human epileptogenic focus. *J. Appl. Physiol.* **4**, 669–676.

Tower, D. B. and MacEachern, D. (1949a). Acetylcholine and neuronal activity. I. Cholinesterase patterns and acetylcholine in the cerebrospinal fluids of patients with craniocerebral trauma. *Can. J. Res.* **27** (Sec. E) 105–119.

Tower, D. B. and MacEachern, D. (1949b). Acetylcholine and neuronal activity. II. Acetylcholine and cholinesterase activity in the cerebrospinal fluids of patients with epilepsy. *Can. J. Res.* **27** (Sec. E) 120–131.

Tuček, S. and Cheng, S. -C. (1970). Precursors of acetyl groups in acetylcholine in the brain *in vivo*. *Biochim. Biophys. Acta* **208**, 538–540.

Uchikawa, H. (1964). Correlation between EEG and cardiovascular effects of adrenaline and some biological peptides. M. Sc. Thesis, Université de Montreal, pp. 40–45.

Ungerstedt, U., Butcher, L. L., Andén, N. -E. and Fuxe, K. (1969). Direct chemical stimulation of dopaminergic mechanisms in the neostriatum of the rat. *Brain Res.* **14**, 461–471.

Vaillant, G. E. (1967). A comparison of antagonists of physostigmine-induced suppression of behavior. *J. Pharmacol. Exp. Therapeut.* **157**, 636–648.

Valdman, A. V. (1961). "The Pharmacology of Reticular Formation and Synaptic Transmission". Leningrad, p. 432.

204 *Central Cholinergic Systems and Behaviour*

Valdman, A. V. (1963). "Problems of Pharmacology of Reticular Formation and Synaptic Transmission". Leningrad, p. 416.

Valverde, F. (1967). Apical dendritic spines of the visual cortex and light deprivation in the mouse. *Exp. Brain Res.* **3,** 337–352.

Valzelli, L. (1967). Drugs and aggressiveness. In "Advances in Pharmacology", pp. 79–108. (S. Garattini and P. A. Shore, Eds) Vol. V, Academic Press, New York and London.

Várszegi, K. M. and Decsi, L. (1967). Some characteristics of the rage reaction evoked by chemical stimulation of the hypothalamus. *Acta Physiol. Acad. Sci. Hung.* **32,** 61–68.

Velluti, R. and Hernández-Peón, R. (1963). Atropine blockade within a cholinergic hypnogenic circuit. *Exp. Neurol.* **8,** 20–29.

Vernadakis, A. and Burkhalter, A. (1967). Acetylcholinesterase activity in the optic lobes of chicks at hatching. *Nature (Lond.)* **214,** 594–595.

Verney, E. B. (1947). The antidiuretic hormone and the factors which determine its release. *Phil. Trans. Roy. Soc. B.* **135,** 25–106.

Victor, M., Angevine, J. B., Mancall, E. L. and Fisher, C. M. (1961). Memory loss with lesions of hippocampal formation. *Archs. Neurol. (Chic).* **5,** 244–263.

Villarreal, J. E. and Domino, E. F. (1964). Evidence for two types of cholinergic receptors involved in EEG desynchronization. *Pharmacologist* **6,** 192.

Vincent, J. D. and Hayward, J. N. (1970). Activity of single cells in the osmoreceptor-supraoptic nuclear complex in the hypothalamus of the waking rhesus monkey. *Brain Res.* **23,** 105–108.

Vinnikov, J. A. and Titova, L. K. (1958). The presence and distribution of specific acetylcholinesterase in the organ of Corti of animals in a state of relative quiet and after exposure to sound. *Dokl. Akad. Nauk SSSR* **119,** 164.

Volkmar, F. R. and Greenough, W. T. (1972). Rearing complexity affects branching of dendrites in the visual cortex of the rat. *Science, N.Y.* **176,** 1445–1447.

Von Baumgarten, R., Bloom, F. E., Oliver, A. P. and Salmoiraghi, G. C. (1963). Response of individual olfactory nerve cells to microelectrophoretically administered chemical sybstances. *Pflüg. Arch. Ges. Physiol.* **277,** 125–140.

von Bechterew, W. V. (1900). Demonstration eines Gehirns mit Zerstörung der vorderen und inneren Theile der Hirnrinde beider Schlafenlappen. *Neurol. Centralbl.* **19,** 990–991.

Votava, Z. (1967). Pharmacology of the central cholinergic synapses. *Ann. Rev. Pharmacol.* **7,** 223–240.

Walker, J. M. (1949). The effect of smoking on water diuresis in man. *Quart. J. Med.* **18,** 51–55.

Walker, J. M. (1957). The release of vasopressin and oxytocin in response to drugs. In "The Neurohypophysis", pp. 229–232. (H. Heller, Ed.) Butterworths, London.

Walsh, R. N., Budtz-Olsen, O. E., Penny, J. E. and Cummins, R. A. (1969). The effects of environmental complexity on the histology of the rat hippocampus. *J. Comp. Neurol.* **137,** 361–365.

Warburton, D. M. and Brown, K. (1972). The facilitation of discrimination performance by physostigmine sulphate. *Psychopharmacologia* **27,** 275–284.

Wasman, M. and Flynn, J. P. (1962). Directed attack elicited from hypothalamus. *Archs. Neurol. (Chic.)* **6,** 220–227.

Wayner, M. J. and Reamanis, G. (1958). Drinking in the rat induced by hypertonic saline. *J. Comp. Physiol. Psychol.* **51,** 11–15.

Weight, F. F. (1968). Cholinergic mechanisms in recurrent inhibition of motoneurons. In "Psychopharmacology: A Review of Progress, 1957–1967", (D. H. Efron, J. O. Cole, J. Levine and J. R. Whittenborn, Eds) U.S. Public Health Service, Publ. No. 1836, pp. 69–75.

Welch, B. L. (1965). Psychophysiological response to the mean level of environmental stimulation: A theory of environmental integration. *In* "Symp. Med. Aspects of Stress in the Military Climate", pp. 39–99, U. S. Govt. Printing Off.,Washington, D.C.

Welch, B. L. (1967). Discussion of the paper on "Aggression, defense and neuro-humors". *Brain Func.* **5,** 150–170.

Welch, B. L. and Welch, A. S. (1968). Greater lowering of brain and adrenal cate-cholamines in group-housed than in individually-housed mice administered DL-α-methyltyrosine. *J. Pharm. Pharmacol.* **20,** 244–246.

Werman, R. (1966). A review—Criteria for identification of a central nervous system transmitter. *Comp. Biochem. Physiol.* **18,** 745–766.

Werman, R. (1972). CNS cellular level: Membranes. *Ann. Rev. Physiol.* **34,** 337–374.

Wetzel, M. C. (1968). Self-stimulation's anatomy: Data needs. *Brain Res.* **10,** 287–296.

Wheatley, M. D. (1944). The hypothalamus and affective behavior. A study of the effects of experimental lesions with anatomic correlations. *Archs. Neurol. Psychiat. (Chic.)* **52,** 296–316.

White, R. P. (1956). Relationship between behavioral changes and brain cholinester-ase activity following graded intracerebral injections of DFP. *Proc. Soc. Exp. Biol. Med.* **93,** 113–116.

White, R. P. (1966). Electrographic and behavioral signs of anticholinergic activity. *Rec. Adv. Biol. Psychiat.* **8,** 127–139.

White, R. P. and Boyajy, L. D. (1959). Comparison of physostigmine and amphet-amine in antagonizing the EEG effects of CNS depressants. *Proc. Soc. Exp. Biol. Med.* **102,** 479–483.

White, R. P. and Daigneault, E. A. (1959). The antagonism of atropine to the EEG effects of adrenergic drugs. *J. Pharmacol. Exp. Therapeut.* **125,** 339–346.

White, R. P., Nash, C. B., Westerbeke, E. J. and Possanza, G. J. (1961). Phylogenetic comparison of central actions produced by different doses of atropine and hyoscine. *Arch. Int. Pharmacodyn.* **132,** 349–363.

White, R. P. and Rudolph, A. S. (1968). Neuropharmacological comparison of sub-cortical actions of anticholinergic compounds. *Progr. Brain Res.* **28,** 14–26.

Whitehouse, L. (1966). The effects of physostigmine on discrimination learning. *Psychopharmacologia* **9,** 183–188.

Whittaker, V. P. (1959). The isolation and characterization of acetylcholine-contain-ing particles from brain. *Biochem. J. (Lond.)* **72,** 694–706.

Whittaker, V. P. (1965). The application of subcellular fractionation techniques to the study of brain function. *Progr. Biophys. Molec. Biol.* **15,** 39–96.

Whittaker, V. P., Michaelson, I. A. and Kirkland, R. J. A. (1964). The separation of synaptic vesicles from nerve ending particles ("synaptosomes"). *Biochem. J. (Lond.)* **90,** 293–303.

Whittier, J. R. and Orr, A. (1962). Hyperkinesia and other physiologic effects of caudate deficit in the adult albino rat. *Neurology (Minneap.)* **12,** 529–539.

Wickelgren, W. A. (1973). The long and the short of memory. *Psychol. Bull.* **80,** 425–438.

Widen, L. and Ajmone-Marsan, C. (1960). Effects of corticipetal and corticifugal impulses upon single elements of the dorsolateral geniculate nucleus. *Exp. Neurol.* **2,** 468–502.

Wiener, N. and Deutsch, J. A. (1968). Temporal aspects of anticholinergic- and anti-cholinesterase-induced amnesia for an appetitive habit. *J. Comp. Physiol. Psychol.* **66,** 613–617.

Wikler, A. (1952). Pharmacological dissociation of behavior and EEG "sleep pattern" in dogs: Morphine, N-allylnormorphine, and atropine. *Proc. Soc. Exp. Biol. Med.* **79**, 261–264.

Willis, W. D. (1971). The case for the Renshaw cell. *Brain Behav. Evolut.* **4**, 5–52.

Wilson, P. D., Pecci-Saavedra, J. and Doty, R. W. (1973). Mesencephalic control of lateral geniculate nucleus in primates. II. Effective loci. *Exp. Brain Res.* **18**, 204–213.

Wilson, V. J. (1959). Recurrent facilitation of spinal reflexes. *J. Gen. Physiol.* **42**, 703–713.

Wilson, V. J. and Burgess, P. R. (1962). Disinhibition in the cat spinal cord. *J. Neurophysiol.* **25**, 392–404.

Wilson, V. J., Diecke, F. P. J. and Talbot, W. H. (1960). Action of tetanus toxin on conditioning of spinal motoneurons. *J. Neurophysiol.* **23**, 659–666.

Winson, J. and Miller, N. E. (1970). Comparison of drinking elicited by eserine or DFP injected into preoptic area of rat brain. *J. Comp. Physiol. Psychol.* **73**, 233–237.

Wolf, G. and Handal, P. J. (1966). Aldosterone-induced sodium appetite: Dose-response and specificity. *Endocrinology* **78**, 1120–1124.

Worden, F. and Livingston, R. (1961). Brain stem reticular formation. *In* "Electrical Stimulation of the Brain", pp. 263–276. (D. Sheer, Ed.) University of Texas Press, Austin.

Yamamoto, C. (1967). Pharmacologic studies of norepinephrine, acetylcholine and related compounds on neurons in Deiters' nucleus and the cerebellum. *J. Pharmacol. Exp. Therapeut.* **156**, 39–47.

Yamamoto, K. and Domino, E. F. (1965). Nicotine induced EEG and behavioral arousal. *Int. J. Neuropharmacol.* **4**, 359–373.

Yamamoto, K. and Domino, E. F. (1967). Cholinergic agonist-antagonist interactions on neocortical and limbic EEG activation. *Int. J. Neuropharmacol.* **6**, 357–373.

Yamashita, H., Koizumi, K. and Brooks, C. M. (1970). Electrophysiological studies of neurosecretory cells in the cat hypothalamus. *Brain Res.* **20**, 462–466.

Zanchetti, A. (1967). Subcortical and cortical mechanisms in arousal and emotional behavior. *In* "The Neurosciences", pp. 602–614. (G. C. Quarton, T. Melnechuk and F. O. Schmitt, Eds) Rockefeller University Press, New York.

Zetler, G. (1968). Cataleptic state and hypothermia in mice, caused by central cholinergic stimulation and antagonised by cholinolytic and antidepressant drugs. *Int. J. Neuropharmacol.* **7**, 325–335.

Zubek, J. P. (Ed.) (1969). "Sensory Deprivation: Fifteen Years of Research". Appleton-Century-Crofts, New York.

Zucker, I. (1971). Light-dark rhythms in rat eating and drinking behavior. *Physiol. Behav.* **6**, 115–126.

# Author Index

Numbers in italics indicate the page on which the reference is listed

## A

Abood, L. G., 5, *167*
Abrahams, V. C., 68, 98, *167*
Adey, W. R., 24, *167*
Aghajanian, G. K., 109, *189, 200*
Agid, R., 48, *193*
Ajmone-Marsan, C., 15, 26, *187, 205*
Albert, D. J., 108, 117, *167, 191*
Allee, W. C., 118, *167, 181*
Allikmets, L. H., 96, *167*
Allmark, M. G., 69, *183*
Altman, J., 120, *167*
Amaro, J., 26, 27, 160, 161, *167, 169, 183*
Anand, B. K., 75, 77, *167, 176*
Anagnoste, B., 44, *182*
Andén, N. E., 29, 37, 44, 58, 59, *167, 203*
Andersson, B., 56, 82, *167*
Angelucci, L., 155, *167*
Angevine, J. B., 108, *203*
Aprison, M. H., 56, 58, *167, 168, 195*
Aquilonius, S. -M., 124, 149, *168*
Ara, R., 162, *186*
Araki, T., 145, *168*
Arango, N. I., 2, 57, *193*
Arbuthnott, G. W., 58, 59, 60, *168*
Arduini, A., 18, 49, *168*
Arduini, M. G., 18, *168*
Arévalo, L., 116, *186*
Arling, G. L., 166, *184*
Armitage, A. K., 65, 124, *168*
Arnfred, T., 36, 140, *168*
Aruguete, A., 5, *195*
Atkinson, K. S., 65, *197*
Austin, L., 54, *168*
Avery, D. D., 73, 98, *168*

## B

Bailey, C. J., *193*
Baker, W. W., 4, 37, 40, 41, 42, 43, 50, 51, 97, 98, 99, *168, 174, 190*

Balázs, R., 48, 49, 117, *168*
Bales, P. D., 5, 56, *185*
Bandler, R. J., 88, 97, 98, 99, 101, 102, 103, *168, 169*
Baratti, C. M., 116, *186*
Barbeau, A., 37, 58, *169*
Barerra, E., 85, *188*
Bargmann, W., 70, *169*
Barker, J. L., 69, 71, *169*
Barker, L. A., 160, 161, *169*
Barros, A., 49, *183*
Bartlett, J. R., 132, *169, 178*
Bartolini, A., 13, 19, 25, 29, 32, 38, 107, 123, 124, 125, 126, 127, 128, 136, 140, 142, 159, *169, 176, 177, 195, 196*
Bartolini, G., 152, *201*
Bartolini, R., 38, *169*
Basagić, E., 102, *186*
Batini, C., 16, 19, *169*
Battista, A. F., 44, *182*
Baxter, B. L., 93, 97, *169*
Beani, L., 18, 25, 124, 142, 143, 146, 148, 149, 155, *169*
Beckman, A. L., 73, 96, *169*
Bédard, P., 37, 44, 46, 47, *190, 197*
Beleslin, D., 124, 132, 150, 152, 155, *169, 170, 194*
Belluzzi, J. D., 98, 112, *170*
Benedict, F., 50, 51, 97, 98, 99, *168*
Bennett, E. L., 89, 103, 107, 117, 119, 120, 166, *170, 177, 182, 189, 198, 199*
Bennett, T. L., 110, *170*
Bernheimer, H., 48, *170*
Bernstein, J. J., 121, *174*
Bertaccini, G., 25, 26, 131, *176*
Bertels-Meeuws, M. M., 157, 158, *170*
Besch, N. F., 82, *170*
Besmedt, J. E., 26, *170*
Bexton, W. H., 166, *170*
Bhatt, R. H. V., 124, *198*
Bhattacharya, B. K., 150, *170*

207

U

Uchikawa, H., 142, *203*
Ungerstedt, U., 29, 32, 37, 58, 59, 107, *167*, *181*, *203*
Unna, K. R., 27, *176*
Urban, I., 72, *194*
Uyeno, E., 119, *197*

V

Vahing, V. A., 96, *167*
Vaillant, G. E., 103, *203*
Valdman, A. V., 21, *203*
Valverde, F., 120, *203*
Valzelli, L., 88, 119, *175*, *181*, *203*
Van Dyne, G. C., 82, *170*
Van Rossum, M. J., 58, 59, *175*
Van Woert, M. H., 109, *200*
Várszegi, K. M., 93, 97, 100, *176*, *203*
Velluti, R., 96, 99, *203*
Vernadakis, A., 119, *203*
Verney, E. B., 70, *203*
Verster, F. De B., 49, *183*
Verzeano, M., 18, *181*
Victor, M., 108, *203*
Villarreal, J. E., 17, *203*
Vincent, J. D., 70, *184*, *203*
Vinnikov, J. A., 27, *203*
Vogt, M., 28, 54, 65, 68, 150, *180*
Volkmar, F. R., 120, *203*
Von Baumgarten, R., 28, *204*
Von Bechterew, W. V., 108, *204*
Voorhoeve, P. E., 56, *175*
Vos, J., 161, *189*
Votava, Z., 3, *204*

W

Wada, S. A., 109, *192*
Walker, C. A., 90, 91, 92, *181*
Walker, J. M., 69, *171*, *204*
Walsh, R. N., 120, *204*
Wanderlinder, L., 26, 27, *167*
Wang, C. -C., 68, *174*
Wang, K. -J., 68, *174*
Warburton, D. M., 116, *204*
Wasman, M., 101, *204*
Watkins, J. C., 33, 35, *176*
Watson, R. H. J., 4, 103, *199*
Watt, J. A., 68, 96, 98, *178*, *197*
Wayner, M. J., 82, *204*

Weight, F. F., 35, *204*
Weisenthal, L. M., 13, 25, 123, 124, 136, *169*
Weiser, H., 48, *185*
Weiss, T., 116, *173*
Welch, A. S., 120, *204*
Welch, B. L., 88, 118, 120, 121, 166, *204*
Werman, R., 123, *204*
Wersall, J., 27, *185*
Westerbeke, E. J., 29, 149, *204*
Westerman, R. A., 152, *192*
Wetzel, M. C., 113, *204*
Wheatley, M. D., 77, 101, *204*
White, C. S., 78, 80, 81, 88, *190*
White, L. E., Jr., 121, *174*
White, R. P., 5, 21, 29, 58, 98, 140, 149, *204*, *205*
Whitehouse, L., 116, *205*
Whitlock, D. G., 14, *195*
Whittaker, V. P., 3, 56, 160, 162, *173*, *186*, *205*
Whittier, J. R., 40, *205*
Wickelgren, W. A., 117, *205*
Widen, L., 26, *205*
Widhalm, S., 48, *191*
Wiener, N., 116, *205*
Wikler, A., 2, 23, 24, *203*, *205*
Willer, H., 97, 110, *183*
Willis, W. D., 36, *205*
Wilson, P. D., 132, *169*, *178*, *205*
Wilson, V. J., 33, 34, 56, *175*, *205*
Wilson, W. C., 4, 72, 96, *185*
Winbladh, B., 124, 149, *168*
Winson, J., 79, 98, *205*
Wirecki, T. S., 65, 100, *172*
Witoslawski, J. J., 105, 112, *184*
Wolf, G., 81, *205*
Wolf, H. H., 74, *199*
Wolfe, L. S., 117, 131, *179*, *201*
Wolstencroft, J. H., 10, 152, 153, *171*, *172*
Woonton, G. A., 49, *194*
Worden, F., 9, *205*
Worzniak, J. J., 4, 61, *181*
Wright, S., 33, *200*
Wycis, H. T., 36, *201*

Y

Yabe, T., 52, *195*
Yaksh, T. L., 73, 74, 81, 88, 91, 96, *194*
Yamamoto, C., 10, *205*

Yamamoto, K., 17, 18, 19, 20, 21, 23, 100, *178*, *205*
Yamamoto, K. I., 17, 23, 100, *177*
Yamashita, H., 70, *205*
Yim, G. K. W., 39, *173*
York, D. H., 2, 15, 134, 152, *196*
Yoshida, H., 161, *192*

Z

Zanchetti, A., 16, 19, 93, 94, *169*, *206*
Zetler, G., 29, 74, *206*
Zornetzer, S. F., 121, *174*
Zubek, J. P., 166, *206*
Zucker, I., 89, *206*

# Subject Index

Renshaw cells, 4, 34–36, 156
Respiratory mechanisms, 4, 61–63
Reticular activating system, 7–16
Reticulo-cortical system, 14, 33
Reticular formation, 4, 7, 9, 10, 12, 15, 23, 24, 26, 94, 110–112, 125, 130
  mesencephalic (MRF), 9, 14, 15, 23, 24, 28, 110, 111, 129
Riboflavin 39, 48
  in globus pallidus, 36

S

Sedatives and hypnotics
  ethyl alcohol, 124
  chlordiazepoxide, 112
  chloral hydrate, 124
  chloralose, 124
  pentobarbital, 112, 124, 146, 148
Self-stimulation behaviour, 112–117
  effect of amphetamine, 115
  effect of antiChE agents, 113
  effect of muscarinic agonists, 114–115
  effect of nicotinic agonists, 115
  role of ACh, 116–117
Septal nuclei, 30
Septum, 31, 78, 82, 85, 93, 113
  in learning and memory, 107–110
Spinal reflexes
  cholinergic nature, 33–36
  recurrent inhibition, 34–36
  Renshaw cells, 4, 34–36
Supraoptic nuclei, 66–72
Substantia nigra, 36, 38, 43, 44, 45, 58, 59, 60
Sympathomimetic amines
  amphetamine, 29, 32, 115, 129, 140, 142, 147, 148
  methamphetamine, 60

T

Tegmentum, 93, 101, 115

Temperature regulation, 4, 72–74
  effect of cholinergics, 74
  effect of tubocurarine, 73
  hypothalamic control
    role of acetylcholine, 72–74
    role of 5-HT, NA, ADR, 72
Tetraethyl pyrophosphate, 61–62
Tetrodotoxin, 128, 144, 145
Thalamic nuclei, 7, 14, 15, 23
Thalamus, 28, 43, 93, 148
Tranquilizers
  chlorpromazine, 60, 103, 112, 148, 151
  haloperidol, 29, 58
  perphenazine, 112
Tremor induced by
  anti-cholinesterases, 37
  cholinergics, 36, 40–41
  muscarinics, 37, 51
  oxotremorine, 36–40
Tremor inhibited by
  hemicholinium-3, 36, 40
Tremor regulating mechanism, 36, 37
Tremor, rest (RT), 36
  cholinergic mechanisms, 36, 43
  dopaminergic mechanisms, 37, 43, 44, 45, 46, 48
  extrapyramidal system, 36
  globus pallidus, 36, 38, 39, 40
  histochemical studies, 43–48

V

Vasopressin (ADH), 4, 68–72
  hypothalamic control, 67–68
  potentiation by ADR, 68
  release by ACh, 4, 68
Ventromedial nuclei, 65–66, 75, 77, 80, 81, 84

Z

Zona incerta, 113

**DATE DUE**

AP 26 78   MY 1 8

DEMCO 38-297